RAPID

WEIGHT LOSS HYPNOSIS

Increase Your Motivation And Self-Esteem With 70 Weekly Positive Affirmations.
A Practical Way To Extreme Weight Loss Through Guided Meditation.

Millennium Wellness Academy

© Copyright 2021 - All rights reserved.

TABLE OF CONTENTS

Introduction

What is weight loss hypnosis?

It's basically using hypnosis techniques to allow you to lose weight. It's a way to shed a few extra pounds. But most of the time, it is paired with a diet plan. It is advisable that you continue a good regimen of food, followed by moderate exercise. But, this will allow you to lose weight faster, and if you're a person who has cravings for things, then this will help you immensely.

It's also a part of the counseling that some people get. You'll be able to get help on your issues regarding food, and this form of hypnosis will allow you to have a better time with your cravings. You can do this with a professional, but you can also do it on your own. It'll allow you to be in control of your life, and you'll control those bad cravings you have.

How it Works

How it works is simple. When you're using hypnosis, you're in a state of absorption and concentration. You're also in a very relaxed and suggestible state, so whatever is said to you is basically taken in a literal manner. You will use mental images to convey the meaning of the words that are said. You'll have your attention focused on that, and when your mind is in a state of concentration, you'll start to have your subconscious handle your cravings. It's a remarkable way to keep yourself in check, and you'll be able to lose a few extra pounds while still trying to keep your body in shape. It's best if you do this with a diet and exercise routine, for it'll allow you to get through it better and achieve more results.

It's best to do this when you have a window of time ready for you to take care of this issue. You'll want at least thirty minutes of quiet time to handle these cravings, ideally an hour at most. You will be handling some pretty heavy matters, so making sure that you're relaxed and able to come back to reality before and after the hypnosis will make it all the better.

Does it Work?

The effectiveness varies from person to person. It will help you, and, on average, a person loses about six pounds. You might lose more, but you might not lose as much as expected. If you're trying to lose a ton of weight, this might not help. But, if you're looking to help eliminate cravings in your life and live a healthier lifestyle, then this is definitely the right tool for you. It's a way to help you supplement your exercising plans, and with this, you'll be able to have an even better time when it comes to shedding those pounds fast.

The Benefits

There are other benefits of using hypnosis for weight loss. The obvious big one is that you lose weight. That's the one people will notice. You'll start to shed those pounds, and you might lose more than you expected. It won't be significant, such as like fifty pounds or more, but if you want to help your body and allow yourself the benefits of being able to control the cravings to lose weight, then this is perfect for you.

Another benefit that people don't realize is how relaxed you are. You'll actually be able to become more relaxed as a result of this. By relaxing the body, you'll be able to also reduce your blood pressure levels and even stop the risk of heart disease. Hypnosis for weight loss allows you to put yourself in a relaxed state for at least an hour, and when you wake up, you'll feel more relaxed. It can also help with bodily tissues, such as muscle aches and pains. If you want to use this to help with those issues as well, it'll definitely do the trick.

Then there are the lasting benefits of it. These are the benefits that you'll get because of the hypnosis. When you're doing this, you'll be able to tackle those parts of your subconscious that think it's okay to eat when you're stressed, or it'll tell you to eat more than necessary. Sometimes, your mind can be your own worst enemy, and this is certainly one of those times. With hypnosis for weight loss, you'll allow yourself to handle your body in a positive manner. If you do this, you'll actually allow yourself to control your cravings and desires through the use of hypnosis. It might seem crazy, but it is possible. It's a great way to take life by the horns, and by doing this, you'll be able to allow yourself the benefit of controlling the factors in your life, such as stress or how much you eat, and turning them around to give yourself a more positive image that will benefit you in ways you've never expected before.

If you're the type of person who wants to change your life and your way of thinking to live a healthier life, then hypnosis for weight loss is perfect for you. With this technique, you'll be targeting different parts of the body, and by doing this, you'll be able to have a much better time when it comes to getting rid of the excess weight. It's a great way to lose weight, and by the end of it, you'll be happier, and the scale will look like a friend, instead of an enemy.

Chapter 1

Mind and Weight loss

Your mind holds the key to your life. You can either let your mind drive you to happiness or malcontent. The good news is that you have the power to reprogram your subconscious mind to lead the life you desire. When you were younger, your mind was a blank slate; it did not have any existing ideas, beliefs, or interpretation of events. Every time someone said something to you, the subconscious absorbed it and stored it away for reference. For example, if you were called fat, worthless, ugly, embarrassing, all that negative information stored away because the mind is always listening and always impartial.

Now that you are older and know better, you believe that it is merely a matter of getting rid of the false notions that your subconscious took hold of in your childhood and youth. It is easier said than done because the subconscious does not respond to the conscious mind. This is because your programming makes decisions for you. Take, for instance; you start a workout routine or a new diet. Your old programming reverts you to your old habits, and you fail miserably at your set goals. This habit can annoy and frustrate you almost forcing you to abandon the quest for a healthier lifestyle. Before you embark on programming your mind to your slim body, keep in mind that you are already that person that you intend to become. You need to develop the capacity to find them within yourself. To learn how to reprogram your mind successfully, you must:

Make A Decision

Decide on the exact outcome you wish for yourself. With clarity comes the power to shape your subconscious in the new paths to follow. Once you have settled on what you want for yourself at this moment and in the future, you are offering your mind resources toward the fulfillment of your objectives. Write it down.

Let's say you want to be 17-pounds lighter by summer three months away. That is a clear-cut objective which you have set for yourself. Put it down clearly on paper, place it within sight so you can see it as often as possible.

Therefore when "external" forces try to sway you into say, indulging or binge eating, you remember that you have set a goal. You have decided to shed seventeen pounds in three months. All of your mental power is aligned to help you accomplish this task.

Commit

Once you have made a clear decision, commit to sticking by it. Commitment means allowing the decision to inform your choices. You may, however, expect to encounter fear. Fear is the biggest threat to success. The fear of failure drives people into giving up on their dreams- not failure itself.

Fear can lead to procrastination of your goals, which in turn feed the fear with negative thoughts such as, "I am better off not trying" or "Why should I risk disappointment in case I fail?" These thoughts cause you to feel even worse than you did before. The best solution for fear is facing it.

Failure is not the end of everything; it is a lesson in itself. Access the first trial, everything you did and how you did it. Examine if there is a way to modify the exercise to alter the result. Therefore, fear should not hold you back from your goals. Your efforts should be coupled with a commitment to a healthier lifestyle, devotion to overcoming the negative thoughts, and above all, commitment to yourself.

Modify Progress

Allow flexibility in your mental capacity. When you have committed to your decision, check the progress to see what is working and what can be amended. Striking a balance between alteration and overhaul can be difficult if you do not have a guide- be it a plan or a mentor or sponsor.

Do not limit yourself to "It's my way or the highway" mentality. Having a peripheral vision can direct you to alternative possibilities and opportunities in case problems arise during your course. Adjusting your programming to cater to these speedbumps builds your resilience to challenges. Your subconscious develops a winning attitude where failures become lessons, hurdles become catapults, and change becomes inevitable.

Overcoming Limitations

To overcome limiting beliefs, you must first acknowledge them and accept them for what they are and the role they have played in your life to this crucial point. The reason it is of significant importance to accept them is that you cannot change what does not exist. These beliefs are repeated to us by society causing us to relate negatively with ourselves, with food, money, and others.

When you realize that these beliefs do not define your worth, you will start to see your true potential and develop self-confidence in your abilities. You will feel free to win at everything in which you set your mind.

Note Down Your Personal Limiting Beliefs

While getting rid of all your limitations, write down the beliefs that you have had from childhood that simply do not serve your purpose anymore. For example, "I am overweight" or "I do not

RAPID WEIGHT LOSS HYPNOSIS

look as good as my petite friends." Such beliefs have likely caused you to look upon yourself with disdain. The negative "I am" thoughts are not honestly what you think of yourself unless someone said them to you.

Understand Causality

The circumstances you find yourself in are not the cause of your limiting beliefs but the effect. Let us take an example of struggling with weight; the reason you are "struggling" is because of your limiting beliefs about food and yourself. Knowing this, you can alter your mentality about your limitations and flip them to work for you instead of against you.

Along with learning how to reprogram our mind, it is essential to note that the subconscious is still taking in new information and using it for reference for future decisions. There are several ways to reprogram your mind successfully.

Environment

The environment that surrounds us impresses significantly on our minds. Imagine if you always have people talking down at you at work or school. That kind of negativity can lead to a host of psychological problems, including depression.

Remove yourself from toxic environments; the instance you start to notice a pattern of ill-intentioned thoughts. Immerse yourself into an environment that fosters loving and positive thoughts. This way, your mind will absorb all the kind thoughts and gradually begin to reprogram your thought pattern. Support groups are an excellent environment to immerse yourself into because not only are these people working with the same set of circumstances, but some have also succeeded in daily progress. They know how rough it can be; therefore, they are the best reference for guidance and support.

Visualization

Visualization is a powerful reprogramming tool. Try to envision your transformed self in day-to-day activities. Envision your perfect romantic life, professional life, family relationships, financial relationships, as well as how you relate to yourself. See yourself as you would like to lead your life and allow yourself to feel fulfilled in these visions.

When these images are accompanied by emotions of accomplishment, gratitude, and joy, the more effectively they will redraw on your earlier images. Your subconscious will see these images as the truth and will guide your decisions based on the repetitive visualization of the images, as mentioned earlier.

For creative visualization to work, you must first change the underlying negative beliefs. This is because the subconscious, being the autopilot, corrects the shift in course whenever you seem to deviate from the norm. Ignoring the limiting beliefs can, by all means, curtail your efforts at reaching your objectives. Address the underlying cause first or use the mental by-product focus method to attaining what you want. This method allows you to focus on something that you do not have negative thoughts about, and therefore, by association helps you achieve what you desire. For example, you may want to travel abroad for summer vacation. You have been saving up for this trip, and you are looking forward to it. By visualizing your perfect self in your ideal trip will enable you to take necessary steps to shred the undesired 17-pounds.

Affirmations

Affirmations are necessary when you want to focus on another thought pattern. During affirmations, you phrase your statements positively, attach personal meaning to them, and repeat them to yourself multiple times throughout the day. Corresponding emotion helps the subconscious to understand the statements and believe them as the new status quo.

At first, getting your conscious mind on board with affirmations that may seem far-fetched can be difficult. As time goes on, however, the power of these affirmations has taken root into your subconscious, and you start to believe them to be true even with your rational mind.

Act as If

This method builds your self-esteem. It works in the same manner as affirmations but uses actions instead of thoughts and words. It is the equivalent of "fake it till you make it" mode of thinking. While your conscious mind is busy judging you about your deceiving mannerisms, your subconscious is loyally picking up on all the subtle differences in thought and sensation as you fake your way to your desired objective.

Actively changing your behaviors causes a change in habits, and sooner, your entire narrative will change.

Hypnosis

Hypnosis is another tool used to reprogram the mind where the hypnotherapist puts you in a state of complete relaxation and reaches into the subconscious mind. Afterward, messages of empowerment and self-reliance are delivered repetitively to the listener. Hypnosis is used to reprogram the self-defeating habits and thoughts that keep you from achieving your goals.

This technique uses creative metaphors, illustrations, and suggestions to rewire the brain. In the wake of hypnosis weight loss studies, women who participated in hypnosis lost twice as much weight as the women who merely watched what they ate. The research, however, is not enough to be conclusive.

The best way to effect hypnosis is to play the messages when you are retiring for the day. As you are about to fall asleep, play the hypnosis tape, and let it carry your mind forward. Doing this in your sleep is more effective because there are limited to no distractions of the conscious mind chatter. The subconscious, being the sponge, absorbs the new thought patterns and rewrites the societal limitations formerly held.

Chapter 2

What Does The Mind Work

The different experiences that you encounter in life are not always sudden and because of your good or back luck, however you choose to define it. Those experiences are a manifestation of your thoughts and feelings, and no matter how much you deny it, your subconscious mind does have quite a role to play in that. Intrigued?

Your intrigue here is legit, but it also shows how oblivious you are to your own power; a power locked inside you waiting for you to tap into it. A power so strong that it can beautifully transform your life, and a power that has been given to you so you live an empowered life.

This power is possessed by your subconscious mind and while many people believe it to be something you cannot unleash, it is quite a doable task and just requires you to comprehend how your mind functions.

The Conscious, Unconscious and Subconscious Minds

It is indeed a difficult task to define explicitly the subconscious mind as your conscious and subconscious minds are most interplaying and may feel to you as one.

Your mind functions on 3 main levels. Your conscious mind is the state that you actively use when you do anything with full awareness. It is what you put to use when you are actively participating in a conversation, while reading, cooking and doing anything else with complete consciousness.

While your conscious mind is in charge of things you do with complete awareness, the truth is you aren't always working with 100% consciousness. Your mind does function on autopilot and if you observe the way you carry out many of your tasks, you will realize that several times, you function mechanically.

For instance, when driving a car, you may unintentionally apply the brakes when it is time to stop at a red traffic signal. While you are consciously seeing the traffic light turn red, your foot automatically hits the brake pedal without you even making that decision consciously.

Similarly, when you enter your house, you may unconsciously leave your shoes out at the door, change into your house slippers and close the door behind your back. You may then move towards your bathroom and put dirty clothes in the laundry as you do every single day.

You are so accustomed to this routine that you may not realize what tasks you engage in consciously. Only when you go through the list with complete attention that you acknowledge what you have been doing.

While you work on these tasks in the present moment, you may not be present while doing them. This happens because your subconscious mind has made you nurture habits of these tasks and makes you function on autopilot to save your time, energy and effort.

Your conscious mind engages in activities based on the efforts of your unconscious and subconscious minds, which are the other two states your mind operates in. Your unconscious mind stores all the information you have picked on over the years including all your fears, all the things you have tasted, every interaction you have had and everything else in between.

Your unconscious mind is indeed a huge storehouse of information and to prevent information overload, your subconscious mind picks out the most important memories and information based on how emotionally involved you were in certain situations, how much you repeat certain instances and how much something means to you.

It stores the recently formed memories and creates a program of how you should work based on all the information locked in your unconscious mind. If you were fond of balloons when you were young and have been buying balloons regularly since then, your subconscious mind makes you nurture a fondness towards balloons. If you have been drinking a glass of water regularly since you were 12, your subconscious mind picks up that information and uses it to create that habit.

Likewise, it picks the beliefs, ideas, viewpoints, fears, inhibitions, doubts and sentiments you strongly believe in and then uses them to build your program. If you have been smoking for a while and feel it helps you cope with stress, your subconscious will make you nurture that belief.

That said, if you think you can overcome any addiction you have, you will have precisely that belief and you will have quite a strong willpower courtesy of that belief and the program created by your subconscious mind based on it.

Throughout the day, your subconscious collects data and sorts through it to check if you need it at any time in the future. It stores information for some time and if you don't come back looking for it, It then tosses it out in the unconscious mind. Every piece of information you have ever picked up on is in your unconscious mind and if you wish to dig it out, you can do so by putting your subconscious mind to use.

The Power of the Subconscious Mind

To succeed in life, do things you aspire to do, manifest all your ambitions and push yourself to do your best, all you need to do is to harness the subconscious mind's power.

While you cannot control all the external factors and events, you encounter, you can definitely control and manage your thoughts and your perception of events and it is this perception that helps you turn even the most unfavorable events to your favor.

Your subconscious as already stated above builds your internal program, which makes you react and respond to different things in different ways. When it picks up from your unconscious mind that you have mostly chickened out of doing things that feel tough for you, it makes you nurture the belief that you cannot overcome your fears.

It is important to point out that your thoughts travel out in the universe and draw towards them other thoughts vibrating on a similar frequency. Everything in the universe is composed of energy and has a certain vibration that it exudes at all times. Things that share a similar vibration are drawn towards one another, which is why the saying goes 'like attracts like.'

Yes, even we human beings exude a certain energy and vibration, which is through our thoughts, emotions and feelings. These feelings and thoughts travel out in the universe and interact with other thoughts and emotions. Those that vibrate at a similar frequency then mingle and are drawn towards each other.

Every thought is accompanied by a host of events, experiences, ideas, concepts and people associated with them. Hence, when a couple of thoughts interact, they bring closer all the other factors and elements associated with them.

When you come across someone at a social situation who is as passionate about plantation and is a staunch environmentalist like you, it is because your thoughts and those of that person met somewhere in the universe and had a ball of their own. They then bring you and the other person together because the two of you share the same energy and vibration.

Similarly, everything that you feel is drawn towards you happens because of the thoughts brewed up by your subconscious. All the good experiences you encounter and all the not so happy ones are also brought closer to you by your thoughts.

If you keep thinking about how bad things will happen to you, eventually you will face them. Remember the time when you kept thinking about how terrible your job interview would go and you did end up making a fool of yourself. Also, recall the time when you were sure that you would get your house mortgage approved and even though your credit history was not too good, you knew you had to get it because you had been saving for your house.

Think of other similar events, when you were and were not so positive on certain outcomes. You will be surprised to learn that your confidence and inhibitions did make you experience outcomes according to your expectations.

All of this happens because of the ramifications of your subconscious mind, and if you do wish to change certain outcomes and experiences for yourself, you only need to reprogram this wonderful creation.

Chapter 3

Hypnosis

For over 200 years, individuals have been contemplating and contending about hypnosis, yet science still needs to explain how it really happens completely. We see what an individual is doing under a trance, yet why the individual is doing it isn't obvious. Ultimately, this riddle is a little piece in a lot bigger riddle: how the human personality works. It is far-fetched that specialists within a reasonable timeframe will think of authoritative clarification of the brain, so It is safe to say that the phenomenon of hypnosis will further remain a mystery. Be that as it may, specialists know the general aspects of hypnosis. As such, they have some examples of how it functions. It is a condition of stupor portrayed by serious suggestive, unwinding, and expanded dream. It is unlike sleep since the individual is alert all times. On the other hand, wandering off into fantasy land, or the feeling of "losing yourself" in a film, is generally common. You are completely mindful. However, most of you're the environment around you is blocked out. To the close to avoidance of some other idea, you focus seriously on the current point. In the day by day daze of ordinary life, a conjured-up universe appears to you to some degree genuine as in it completely connects with your feelings. Specific occasions can trigger genuine dread, misery, or satisfaction, and in case you're stunned by something (for instance, a beast hopping out of the shadows), you may even shake in your seat. That is why most analysts characterize every single daze as self-trance of sorts. Milton Erickson, the twentieth century's driving master in sleep induction, contended that people are mesmerized every day. In any case, most specialists focus on the condition of daze brought about by purposeful unwinding and thinking works out. This significant mesmerizing is frequently compared among alertness and rest to the casual mental state.

In a standard trance, as though they were the truth, you approach the trance specialist's recommendations or your considerations. On the off chance that the trance inducer demonstrates your tongue has swollen up to twice its size, you will feel an inclination in your mouth, and you may experience issues talking. In case you're drinking a chocolate milkshake, the trance specialist demonstrates, you'll taste the milkshake and feel it cooling your mouth and throat. If you are frightened, the subliminal specialist shows, you may feel panicky or start perspiring. Yet, constantly, you know it's everything fanciful. As youngsters do, you "play imagining" on an extraordinary level.

Individuals feel uninhibited and agreeable in this specific mental state. This is most likely because they settle the worries and questions that normally hold their exercises under tight restraints. While watching a film, you may encounter a similar impression; as you get inundated in the plot, worries about your work, family, and so on blur away, until all you're considering is what's on the screen.

You're likewise amazingly suggestible in this state. That is, if the subliminal specialist advises you to accomplish something, you are probably going to embrace the idea completely. This is the thing that makes it so agreeable to demonstrate the stage subliminal specialist. Delicate grown-ups are typically held to stroll around the stage all of a sudden, clucking like chickens or singing as loud as possible. There is, by all accounts, the dread of humiliation flying out the window. Nonetheless, the suspicion that all is the well and good and ethical quality of the subject stays installed all through the experience. You can't get a subliminal specialist to do anything you would prefer not to do.

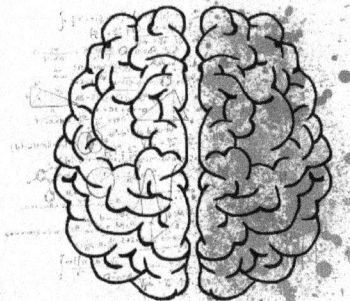

Hypnosis in Psychology

What exactly is hypnosis?

While definitions may contrast, the American Psychological Association characterizes hypnosis as an agreeable collaboration in which the member responds to the hypnotist's recommendations. Because of basic acts, the trance has turned out to be notable where people are urged to direct unprecedented or silly conduct, yet also clinically demonstrated to give medicinal and restorative favorable circumstances, mosquitoes. Hypnosis has even been recommended to diminish dementia manifestations.

What do you think when you hear the term trance specialist? In case you're similar to numerous people, the term may invoke photos of a vile stage miscreant who, by swinging a pocket watch to and fro, makes a sleep-inducing state.

Truth be told, there is little similitude among mesmerizing and these cliché portrayals. "The trance specialist doesn't mesmerize the person, as indicated by analyst John Kihlstrom. Or maybe, the trance specialist fills in as a sort of mentor or coach whose assignment is to help the individual turned out to be mesmerized."

While hypnosis, or even, spellbinding is regularly characterized as a rest, like a dazed state, it is better explained as a condition of concentrated consideration, expanded suggestive and clear dreams. Individuals in a mesmerized state frequently appear to be lethargic and daydreaming, yet they are in a condition of hyper-cognizance truth be told.

Spellbinding is now and then alluded to as hypnotherapy in brain research and has been utilized for a few reasons, including agony abatement and treatment. Ordinarily, trance is finished by a certified specialist who uses perception and verbal reiteration to cause an entrancing condition.

Impacts of Hypnosis

Entrancing knowledge can vary significantly from individual to person. Some spellbound individuals report feeling separation or outrageous unwinding during the mesmerizing state while others even think their exercises have all the earmarks of being occurring outside their cognizant will. Other individuals, while under spellbinding, may remain completely cognizant and ready to lead talks.

Scientist Ernest Hilgard's examinations demonstrated how spellbinding could be utilized to drastically change discernments. The member's arm was then placed in ice water in the wake of training a mesmerized individual not to feel torment in their arm while individuals who were not spellbound needed to expel their arm from the water.

Where is Hypnotism Utilized?

Through research, spellbinding has been utilized in the treatment of different conditions, for example,

- Alleviating constant excruciating conditions like rheumatoid joint pain

- Alleviating and treating torment in labor

- Reducing dementia side effects

- For some ADHD side effects, hypnotherapy might be of assistance

- Reducing the impacts of sickness prompting retching in disease patients on chemotherapy

- Reducing torment when experiencing a dental technique

- Improving and taking out skin conditions, for example, psoriasis and moles

- Reducing touchy inside disorder manifestations

So, for what reason should an individual endeavor in spellbinding? In certain examples, people might search for entrancing to help constant agony or ease torment and nervousness brought about by restorative procedures, for example, medical procedure or birth.

Mesmerizing has likewise been utilized to help people with conduct changes, for example, smoking end, weight reduction, or bed-wetting counteractive action.

Is it possible to hypnotize yourself?

While numerous people accept that they can't be hypnotized, a study has demonstrated that numerous individuals are more hypnotizable than they might suspect.

- Fifteen percent of people are profoundly receptive to spellbinding.

- Children are bound to be inclined to spellbinding.

- It is respected hard or difficult to spellbind around 10% of grown-ups.

- People who can ingest themselves promptly in dreams are substantially more receptive to spellbinding.

If you are keen on being mesmerized, moving toward the involvement with a receptive outlook is basic to recall. Research has proposed that individuals who take a good viewpoint of mesmerizing will, in general, respond better.

Chapter 4

Self-Hypnosis

The only significant difference between hypnosis and self-hypnosis is that in the first one, the operator and the subject are two different people, while in self-hypnosis the operator and the subject coincide in the same person.

It can be very positive to share the self-hypnosis learning experience with another person using the methods described in this volume. This shared experience can be of great value to both, as it will unite them mentally and emotionally and promote love and mutual respect.

It is also a fact that learning is easier and faster when done with another person.

Ask your partner to hypnotize you using a procedure similar to the one we used in the second session. Then practice the self-hypnosis exercise for a few days. Ask your partner once again to hypnotize you and reinforce hypnotic suggestion. Practice it again.

The number of times it is necessary to reinforce the procedure depends entirely on you. If you practice the daily self-hypnosis exercise, one or two reinforcement sessions will be sufficient.

But what about those who have no one with whom to share the learning experience of self-hypnosis? What can they do? How can they learn?

Leave your worries aside.

It is possible to use self-hypnosis to solve virtually any type of problem and also to broaden your consciousness and connect with your innate superior intelligence and creative ability. By using self-hypnosis for the latter purpose, hypnosis can be transformed into meditation.

Self-hypnosis can also be used in those moments when you feel the need for a higher power to intervene in some situations; Then, it becomes a prayer. The subtle differences between these forms of self-hypnosis lie in the way thoughts are guided once the state of consciousness itself has been altered, that is when the alpha state has been reached.

Then I will tell you a fun experience that happened to me with self-hypnosis. I had an appointment with the dentist to have two molars removed. Last night I had conditioned myself to stop the flow of blood.

On the day of the appointment, when sitting in the dentist's chair, I self-reported. When the dentist removed the teeth, I blocked the flow of blood so that it did not flow through the open wound. The dentist was perplexed and kept telling his assistant: «It doesn't bleed.

How is it possible?. I don't understand it. I smiled mentally since I couldn't physically smile because of all the devices, cotton, and other objects that held my mouth. Also, I visualized quick and complete healing. After seventy-two hours the swelling had subsided, and the wounds had healed completely;

And now, I will tell you another funny experience that one of my patients had with self-hypnosis.

He was part of a group that participated in an investigation about dreams at the local hospital. Once a week, my patient slept in the hospital with an electroencephalogram (EEG) connected to his head. This was intended to record the waves of their brain activity.

By observing the graph, doctors could establish if they were an alpha, beta, tit, or delta state, and they could also state when the patient was sleeping and when he was awake. My client immediately hypnotized himself as soon as he was connected to the EEG.

The apparatus recorded a deep alpha state, indicative that the subject was sleeping, although he was fully awake. One of the doctors asked: "What's going on here?" Then the man alternately returned to the beta state, then to alpha, then again to beta, and finally to alpha while the machine registered it.

The changes confused the doctors until the subject told them what he was doing. The response of the doctors cannot be reproduced here.

What does this mean?. It means that it is possible to develop an activity and keep your eyes open even if one is in an altered state of consciousness. Think about it for a moment.

What a wonderful tool is self-hypnosis! It transports us to another state while we are comfortably and quietly sitting with our eyes closed, thinking about a specific objective. But using self-hypnosis in this sense is not easy to achieve since it requires a prolonged period of preconditioning in a hypnotic or autohypnotic state. Such preconditioning is similar to that used for diet control, but the indications are different; It will be necessary to devise the techniques and suggestions for this case.

And it also requires practice, a lot of practice. Do not forget my words, time and effort will be rewarded with the results. Develop your discipline and stick to it; The results will be a real success.

Where to Practice Hypnosis

It can be practiced anywhere, including dimly lit rooms, sunny exteriors, quiet places, and noisy places. However, the ideal place is a comfortable and quiet room with soft lighting.

If unexpected distractions take place, you should use them to your advantage. I had just started a hypnosis session when a carpenter began riveting nails in the following office, right on the wall behind my patient's head. I abandoned the usual hypnotic induction exercise and began to improvise. Outside noises do not distract you. On the contrary, they will help you reach the healthiest state of relaxation. Then, with each hammer, he said: Relax more deeply (bang); more deeply (bang); more and more deeply (bang). My patient went into deep relaxation as if he had been in an elevator that was descending at high speed. It was not even necessary to continue with the rest of the exercises, I just verbalized the suggestions and then returned it to its conscious state. The results were excellent.

Hypnosis During Sleep

There is yet another very effective use of hypnosis that is easy to put into practice: falling asleep listening to a tape that you will have formerly recorded. I am not referring to using hypnosis to sleep better - although it is also possible to use it for that purpose - but to apply it to achieve any goal you set.

Neither your subconscious mind nor your auditory faculties ever sleep. Therefore, even if you are asleep as the tape progresses, your brain absorbs all the information and begins the process of materializing your reality. When you sleep, you are in a deep hypnotic state, and for this reason, the procedure is very useful. Perform the following three steps:

1. Record the exercises A, B, C, D, E, F, I, G, U, and V and then verbalize everything you want to come true.

2. When you decide to go to sleep, connect the recorder.

3. This will automatically disconnect at the end of the tape without you waking up.

Display instructions are not included in the tapes used for this procedure, only verbal indications. The method is very useful. For example, suppose you have a job interview the following day. In this case, you will include in the tape the appropriate suggestions to succeed in said interview. You will be serene, you will speak intelligently, you will be attentive without being effusive, and so on. Then you will go to sleep while the tape does all the work. The following day the interview will be a success.

Physical Position During Hypnosis

It can be practiced standing or sitting. Patients can rest on a comfortable sofa, sit in a straight-backed chair, lie on a bed or on the floor, sit cross-legged, or stand. All positions are correct, but not necessarily for all situations. For example, a brief two-minute procedure aimed at eliminating pain is suitable for a person who is standing. Still, a thirty-minute method that aims to control diet cannot be practiced with a patient who remains standing.

A reclining chair or straight backrest, or a chair without armrests, are the most suitable for this situation since they offer the subject adequate support and are comfortable; Also, it will be difficult for the subject to fall asleep sitting in any of these chairs. I prefer that my patients use a reclining chair. However, when I practice self-hypnosis, I opt for a straight back chair without armrests. As an operator, I also prefer this type of chair.

Lying on a bed is comfortable for the subject, but has the disadvantage that he can fall asleep during the session since both the body and the mind are conditioned to sleep when the individual adopts this position, and the brain reaches alpha. An experienced operator can prevent this from happening. When working with someone bedridden, one should work in this position.

Lying on the floor offers the same inconvenience: the subject will tend to fall asleep. Besides, the soil is usually uncomfortable, and for this reason, I do not recommend it when using long-term procedures.

Sitting cross-legged on the floor is also an awkward position and is not advisable for lengthy procedures. I usually use this position to meditate (a form of self-hypnosis), and I get excellent results. I once remained in deep meditation for an hour and a half in this position without experiencing any physical discomfort. I doubt that an inexperienced person could stay in that position and then be able to stand up and, even less, to start walking.

In general, my patients use the reclining chair, and I stand in front of them in a straight-backed chair. The distance between the two is about 60 centimeters to 1.50 meters. It is completely indifferent that there is a table or a desk between us. I place myself close enough to the subject to speak in a normal tone of voice and to listen to me perfectly, but far enough away not to intimidate him/her. For some procedures that I use on special occasions, I must stand beside the subject or even have physical contact with him/her. This is not the rule but an exception.

Ideally, the subject's chair should be located in such a way that their eyes do not receive light. The windows (unless the curtains are very thick) and the lights should be behind the patient, as this will make it easier to relax and be comfortable.

Chapter 5

Why Hypnosis Can Be
A Solution For Weight Loss

Hypnosis might be best known as the gathering stunt used to make people move the chicken in front of an audience. However, an ever-increasing number of people go to the psychological control system to help them make more beneficial choices and get in shape. A valid example: The consuming fewer calories master changed to spellbinding when Georgia, 28, chose she required to shed the 30 pounds she put on after foot medical procedure in 2009. The technique for mind-control had helped her in the past to conquer a dread of flying, and she trusted that it would likewise enable her to make good dieting practices.

Georgia subsequently decided to engage in hypnotherapy to help her lose weight. In short, each session was focused on planting positive thoughts in her mind such as knowing when to stop eating and finding the best way to help her stop overeating based on emotional reactions. The treatment proved to be progressively effective as she was able to curb her appetite and manage her eating habits more effectively. She was able to drop the weight that she wanted based on improving her overall eating habits, curbing her cravings and limiting the instances of binge eating.

Mesmerizing is for anybody searching for a mellow way to get thinner and make smart dieting a propensity. Is it safe to say that it isn't for one person? Any individual who needs a quick fix. It expects time to reframe issue thoughts regarding sustenance Georgia reveals to her trance inducer eight times each year, and it took a month before she started to see a genuine change. "The weight fell gradually and definitely, without tremendous adjustments in my way of life. I was all the while eating out many times each week, yet regularly sending plates back with sustenance on them! I truly tasted my sustenance unexpectedly, investing energy in flavors and surfaces. It was as though I had begun my illicit affection relationship with nourishment, no one, but I could get thinner," she said.

Spellbinding isn't planned to be a "diet," but instead an apparatus to help you prevail with regards to eating and practicing nutritious sustenance, states Traci Stein, Ph.D., MPH, an ASCH-ensured clinical entrancing wellbeing clinician and former Director of Integrative Medicine at Columbia University's Department of Surgery. "Spellbinding enables people to encounter what they feel when they are ground-breaking, fit, and indirection in a multi-tactile way and conquer their psychological hindrances to accomplish those goals," she guarantees. "In particular, trance can help people unravel the hidden mental issues that reason them to abhor work out, experience extreme longings, gorge during the evening, or eat heedlessly. It empowers them to recognize the triggers and incapacitate them.

"As a general rule, it is valuable not to consider mesmerizing an eating regimen by any stretch of the imagination, says Joshua E. Syna, MA, LCDC, an authorized trance specialist at the Houston Hypnosis Center." It works since it changes their perspective about sustenance and eating and empowers them to figure out how to be increasingly quiet and agreeable in their life. So as opposed to being a passionate answer for sustenance and eating, it turns into a reasonable answer for craving, and new personal conduct standards are being made that enable the person to adapt to sentiments and life, "he depicts." Hypnosis works for weight reduction since it enables the person to isolate nourishment and eat from their enthusiastic lives.

Dr. Stein proposes that utilizing at-home independently directed sound projects produced by a gifted subliminal specialist (search for an ASCH affirmation) is alright for people with no other emotional wellness issues. Be that as it may, be careful with all the new online market applications, one investigation found that most applications are untested and regularly make affected cases about their viability that can't be substantiated.

What Hypnosis Feels Like

Forget what you found in movies and front of an audience is more like a treatment session than a carnival stunt. "Trance is a community-oriented encounter and at all times ought to be very much educated and agreeable," says Dr. Stein.

What's more, she adds to individuals stressed over being fooled into accomplishing something odd or hurtful, even under entrancing on the off chance that you would prefer truly not to accomplish something, you won't. "Consideration is simply focused," she portrays. "Normally everybody goes into light daze articulations a few times each day-accept about when you daydream while a companion shares everything about their vacation and trance just figures out how to think that internal consideration in a supportive way." Dispelling the legend that entrancing feels weird or terrifying from the patient's side, Georgia claims she generally felt exceptionally clear and leveled out.

There were even entertaining occasions such as envisioning steps on the scale and seeing the heaviness of her target. "My excessively inventive personality needed to envision initially taking off all garments, all of the gems, my watch, and barrette before hopping on naked. Any other individual does that, or is it just me?" (No, it's not simply you, Georgia!)

It's not intrusive, it functions admirably with other weight reduction medications, and it doesn't include any pills, powders, or different enhancements. Nothing occurs even from a pessimistic standpoint, placing it in the camp "may help, can't hurt." But Dr. Stein concedes that one drawback is there: cost. Expenses every hour contrast dependent on your place, yet for helpful spellbinding systems, it differs from $100-$250 an hour and when you see the specialist for a month or two once per week or more that can include rapidly. What's more, trance isn't secured by most insurance agencies. Be that as it may, Dr. Stein proposes it very well may be secured whenever utilized as a major aspect of a greater arrangement for psychological wellness treatment, so check with your provider. A surprising perk of weight loss hypnosis isn't only a psychological thing, it's likewise a medicinal component, says Peter LePort, MD, a bariatric specialist, and Memorial Care Center for Obesity's therapeutic chief in California. "You should initially adapt to any hidden metabolic or natural weight increase causes yet utilizing spellbinding can kick start sound propensities while that is no joke," he proposes. Furthermore, there is another great advantage of utilizing spellbinding: "The component of reflection can diminish pressure and lift mindfulness, which can likewise help with weight reduction," he added.

How Hypnosis Aids In Weight Loss

There is an amazing measure of logical research that takes a gander at the viability of weight reduction mesmerizing, and a lot of it is sure. One of the underlying 1986 research found that overweight females utilizing a mesmerizing project shed 17 pounds contrasted with 0.5 pounds for females just advised to watch what they ate. A mesmerizing weight reduction study meta-investigation during the 1990s found that members who utilized trance lost more than twice as much weight as the individuals who didn't. Also, an examination in 2014 found that females who utilized entrancing were improving their weight, BMI, eating conduct, and even certain parts of self-perception.

In any case, it's not all uplifting news: A Stanford study in 2012 found that about a fourth of individuals just can't be mesmerized, and it has nothing to do with their characters, as opposed to basic conviction. Or maybe, the minds of certain individuals simply don't appear to work that way. "In case you're not inclined to staring off into space, you regularly think that it's difficult to stall out in a volume or endure a motion picture, and don't believe you're innovative, you may be one of the individuals for whom trance isn't functioning admirably," says Dr. Stein.

Georgia is one of the examples of overcoming adversity. She guarantees it helped her lose the extra pounds as well as helped her keep them off also. After six years, she kept her weight reduction joyfully, now and then returning in with her trance specialist when she requires a boost.

Chapter 6

Affirmations: An Important And Useful Practice

A ffirmations are a wonderful tool to use alongside hypnosis to help you rewire your brain and improve your weight loss abilities. Affirmations are essentially a tool that you use to remind you of your chosen "rewiring" and to encourage your brain to opt for your newer, healthier mindset over your old unhealthy one. Using affirmations is an important part of anchoring your hypnosis efforts into your daily life, so it is important that you use them on a routine basis.

When using affirmations, it is important that you use ones that are relevant and that are going to actually support you in anchoring your chosen reality into your present reality.

What Are Affirmations, and How Do They Work?

Anytime you repeat something to yourself out loud, or in your thoughts, you are affirming something to yourself. We use affirmations on a consistent basis, whether we consciously realize it or not. For example, if you are on your weight loss journey and you repeat "I am never going to lose the weight" to yourself on a regular basis, you are affirming to yourself that you are never going to succeed with weight loss. Likewise, if you are consistently saying, "I will always be fat" or "I am never going to reach my goals" you are affirming those things to yourself, too. When we use affirmations unintentionally, we often find ourselves using affirmations that can be hurtful and harmful to our psyche and our reality. You might find yourself locking into becoming a mental bully toward yourself as you consistently repeat things to yourself that are unkind and even downright mean. As you do this, you affirm a lower sense of self-confidence, a lack of motivation, and a commitment to a body shape and wellness journey that you do not actually want to maintain.

Affirmations, whether positive or negative, conscious, or unconscious, are always creating or reinforcing the function of your brain and mindset. Each time you repeat something to yourself, your subconscious mind hears it and strives to make it a part of your reality. This is because your subconscious mind is responsible for creating your reality and your sense of identity. It creates both around your affirmations since these are what you perceive as being your absolute truth; therefore, they create a "concrete" foundation for your reality and identity to rest on. If you want to change these two aspects of yourself and your experience, you are going to need to change what you are routinely repeating to yourself so that you are no longer creating a reality and identity rooted in negativity. In order to change your subconscious experience, you need to consciously choose positive affirmations and repeat them on a constant basis to help you achieve the reality and identity that you truly want. This way, you are more likely to create an experience that reflects what you are looking for, rather than an experience that reflects what your conscious and subconscious mind has automatically picked up on. The key with affirmations is that you need to understand that your brain does not care if you are creating them on purpose or not. It also does not care if you are creating healthy and positive ones or unhealthy and negative ones. All your subconscious mind cares about is what is repeated to it, and what you perceive as being your absolute truth. It is up to you and your conscious mind to recognize that negative and unhealthy affirmations will hold you back, prevent you from experiencing positive experiences in life, and result in you feeling incapable and unmotivated. Alternatively, consciously choosing healthy and positive affirmations will help you with creating a mindset that is healthier and an identity that actually serves your wellbeing on a mental, physical, emotional, and spiritual level. From there, your responsibility is to consistently repeat these affirmations to yourself until you believe them, and you begin to see them being reflected in your reality.

How Do I Pick and Use Affirmations for Weight Loss?

Choosing affirmations for your weight loss journey requires you to first understand what it is that you are looking for, and what types of positive thoughts are going to help you get there. You can start by identifying what your dream is, what you want your ideal body to look and feel like, and how you want to feel as you achieve your dream of losing weight. Once you have identified what your dream is, you need to identify what current beliefs you have around the dream that you are aspiring to achieve. For example, if you want to lose 25 pounds so that you can have a healthier weight, but you believe that it will be incredibly hard to lose that weight, then you know that your current beliefs are that losing weight is hard. You need to identify every single belief surrounding your weight loss goals and recognize which ones are negative or are limiting and preventing you from achieving your goal of losing weight.

After you have identified which of your beliefs are negative and unhelpful, you can choose affirmations that are going to help you change your beliefs. Typically, you want to choose an affirmation that is going to help you completely change that belief in the opposite direction. For example, if you think "losing weight is hard," your new affirmation could be "I lose the weight effortlessly." Even if you do not believe this new affirmation right now, the goal is to repeat it to yourself enough that it becomes a part of your identity and, inevitably, your reality. This way, you are anchoring in your hypnosis sessions, and you are effectively rewiring your brain in between sessions, too.

As you use affirmations to help you achieve weight loss, I encourage you to do so in a way that is intuitive to your experience. There is no right or wrong way to approach affirmations, as long as you are using them on a regular basis. Once you feel yourself effortlessly believing in an affirmation, you can start incorporating new affirmations into your routine so that you can continue to use your affirmations to improve your wellbeing overall. Ideally, you should always be using positive affirmations even after you have seen the changes you desire, as affirmations are a wonderful way to help naturally maintain your mental, emotional, and physical wellbeing.

What Should I Do with My Affirmations?

After you have chosen what affirmations you want to use, and which ones are going to feel best for you, you need to know what to do with them! The simplest way to use your affirmations is to pick 1-2 affirmations and repeat them to yourself on a regular basis. You can repeat them anytime you feel the need to re-affirm something to yourself, or you can repeat them continually even if they do not seem entirely relevant in the moment. The key is to make sure that you are always repeating them to yourself so that you are more likely to have success in rewiring your brain and achieving the new, healthier, and more effective beliefs that you need to improve the quality of your life.

In addition to repeating your affirmations to yourself, you can also use them in many other ways. One way that people like using affirmations is by writing them down. You can write your affirmations down on little notes and leave them around your house, or you can make a ritual out of writing your affirmations down a certain amount of times per day in a journal so that you are able to routinely work them into your day. Some people will also meditate on their affirmations, meaning that they essentially meditate and then repeat the affirmations to themselves over and over in a meditative state. If repeating your affirmation to yourself like a mantra is too challenging, you can also say your chosen affirmations to yourself on a voice recording track and then repeat them to yourself on loop while you meditate. Other people will create recordings of themselves repeating several affirmations into their voice recorder and then listening to them on loop while they work out, eat, drive to work, or otherwise engage in an activity where affirmations might be useful.

If you really want to make your affirmations effective and get the most out of them, you need to find a way to essentially bombard your brain with this new information. The more effectively you can do this, the more your subconscious brain is going to pick up on it and continue to reinforce your new neural pathways with these new affirmations. Through that, you will find yourself effortlessly and naturally believing in the new affirmations that you have chosen for yourself.

How Are Affirmations Going to Help Me Lose Weight?

Affirmations are going to help you lose weight in a few different ways. First and foremost, and probably most obvious, is the fact that affirmations are going to help you get in the mindset of weight loss. To put it simply: you cannot sit around believing nothing is going to work and expect things to work for you. You need to be able to cultivate a motivated mindset that allows you to create success. If you are unable to believe that it will come true: trust that it will not come true.

As your mindset improves, your subconscious mind is actually going to start changing other things within your body, too. For example, rather than creating desires and cravings for things that are not healthy for you, your body will begin to create desires and cravings for things that are healthy for you. It will also stop creating inner conflict around making the right choices and taking care of yourself. In fact, you may even find yourself actually falling in love with your new diet and your new exercise routine. You will also likely find yourself naturally leaning toward behaviors and habits that are healthier for you without having to try so hard to create those habits. In many cases, you might create habits that are healthy for you without even realizing that you are creating those habits. Rather than having to consciously become aware of the need for habits, and then putting in the work to create them, your body and mind will naturally begin to recognize the need for better habits and will create those habits naturally as well.

Some studies have also suggested that using affirmations will help your brain and subconscious mind actually govern your body differently, too. For example, you may be able to improve your body's ability to digest things and manage your weight naturally by using affirmations and hypnosis. In doing so, you may be able to subconsciously adjust which hormones, chemicals, and enzymes are created within your body to help with things like digestive functions, energy creation, and other weight- and health-related concerns that you may have.

Chapter 7

Lose Weight Through Guided Meditation

Reducing extra pounds is the problem, perhaps, of every woman who requires a lot of work, courage, patience, and willpower. But often the hours spent on the simulator, strenuous exercises, exhausting hunger strikes do not give the desired result; weight loss does not occur. But many people do not even realize that you can lose weight using a simple and enjoyable way.

This slimming meditation is a simple and natural tool that will help promote progress in weight loss.

Meditation is often seen as a relaxing practice, but one that benefits the mind only, not the body. Indeed, when you think "I have to lose weight," you will tend to see yourself exercising more and dieting. However, the first step in these two methods is basically going through your head. So we will see how we can effectively practice meditation to lose weight.

How Meditation Helps Lose Weight

It would seem that how meditation can help women lose weight? But in fact, meditation practice has many advantages:

- Metabolism regulation. With regular practice, the human body restores its biological functions, including metabolism. This contributes to the fact that weight loss occurs naturally, fat deposits go away. A good metabolism in the body also causes a decrease in appetite, which is why a person eats less.

- Digestion. Meditation helps to improve the absorption of food. Hormonal imbalances in the female body and stress lead to overeating and indigestion. Regular exercise helps relax your nerves and balance hormones. This has a long-term impact on efforts to reduce extra pounds.

- Legibleness in food. One of the biggest obstacles to weight loss is the craving for unhealthy and unhealthy foods. Slimming meditation eliminates these unhealthy urges. A person becomes more attentive to what he eats, as he takes care of his own body and therefore loses weight.

- Stress resistance. Very often, overeating occurs due to stress. Experiencing, a person himself does not notice the growth of his appetite. This leads to a set of extra pounds. That is why meditation is so important for losing weight because it eliminates the primary source of the problem - reduces stress.

- Discipline. Uncontrolled meals and snacks are associated with the fact that a person can not refuse his favorite food. The only way to perfection is faith in oneself, willpower, clarity of mind, and discipline. By meditating regularly, all these qualities can be developed and strengthened in oneself.

- Self-hypnosis. Much is known about the power of thought - they materialize and become a reality if efforts are made. In this case, meditation works like hypnosis - a person programs himself for the result.

How to lose weight while meditating

Meditation on harmony should be a daily practice. For effectiveness, it is recommended to meditate daily for at least 20 minutes.

Slimming meditation does not have to be difficult. If you're a beginner, try starting five minutes in the morning to clear your mind before confronting a busy day and five minutes before going to bed. Yoga instructors note that, in principle, the time of classes does not matter if you meditate regularly and correctly. You can see the results of losing weight only if meditation becomes a habit.

The rules of meditation if you want to lose weight:

- Use a mantra to help you lose weight. A mantra is a word or phrase that you repeat to yourself in order to focus on the goal when your mind wanders. These are words that can eventually enter into meditative hypnosis.

- Watch your breath. Just close your eyes and focus on your breath without trying to change it. If your mind wanders — and it will be so at first — just direct it back to your breath.

- Meditation for excellence in losing weight should not be stressful. In the process, a person should feel comfortable, and this applies to everything: clothing, posture, environment, well-being.

Step-by-step instruction

Anyone who wants to lose weight can meditate. To exercise, there is no need for special equipment or expensive classes. For many, the hardest part is simply finding the time. But on the road to your goal, you can do it.

- Make sure you have the opportunity to create silence for the time you need.

- When you find yourself in a quiet place, calm yourself, relax. You can sit or lie down in any position that is convenient.

- Start by focusing on your breath, observing your chest or stomach when it rises and falls. Feel the air as it moves and exits your mouth or nose. Listen to the sounds that air makes. Do this for a minute or two until you begin to feel more relaxed.

- Then, with your eyes open or closed, do the following: Take a deep breath. Hold it for a few seconds. Exhale slowly and repeat. Inhale naturally. Observe your breathing when it enters your nostrils, raise your chest, or moves your stomach, but do not alter it in any way. Keep focusing your breath for 5-10 minutes.

- Start to visualize. Imagine how you are slim and beautiful, put on your favorite dress, how you walk along the catwalk, how men turn around after you. In weight loss meditation, it is important for women to increase their self-esteem, to understand that change is necessary for the perfection of themselves.

Meditation Results for Weight Loss

If you want to meditate specifically in order to lose weight, look for exercises focused on this. Losing weight meditation looks more like hypnosis or self-hypnosis. It is important to form the power of thought, the power of will. It is important to impress upon yourself that you really want something (to lose weight in this situation) and strive to fulfill your desire.

This can be a visualization of how you can look and feel after you have lost weight. You can imagine yourself slim and thin, mentally put on your favorite clothes.

But with all the benefits of meditation when losing weight, it is only one method in a set of actions for losing weight. It is impossible to lose weight, just meditating. If you eat kilograms of chips and buns and can not reduce your appetite, then even many hours of meditation will not save you and will not help to reduce weight.

Proper nutrition and exercise are also important parts of the path to harmony. There will always be better results if you combine all these components into one and make them your way of life.

Meditative practice, first of all, changes the thinking, consciousness, attitude to the problem, helps to strengthen desire and desire for the goal. Studies show that these changes take only 21 days. It is in three weeks that a person's habits change and form, including eating right and eating little, refusing junk food, and drinking plenty of water - this also helps to lose weight.

As you can see, meditation is the key to harmony, an amazing technique in which there is not a single side effect. This practice can change a person, both internally and physically, for the better.

Benefits of Meditation For Weight Loss

1. Get more energy.

Meditating for three to five minutes a day gives your mind and body a chance to rest, relax, rejuvenate, and refresh your body to every cell.

2. Feel Good.

The better you feel, the easier you'll be to lose the pounds. Instead of grabbing a sweet cake, try meditating for a few minutes until the craving goes away. Try that!

3. Better focus.

The more you meditate, the more you can concentrate. Meditation is also a practice in which specific thoughts are based. The more you can focus, the more you can concentrate on meeting your weight goals.

4. Reduce Stress and Anxiety.

Some people go to the gym to relieve tension, and meditation may take place. Even if you exorcize the body and still have tension, the body still retains all this tension. If the mind holds you back, the body will hold you back. Why not both. Why not.

5. Lose Weight.

The physiology of the body is usually such that what we do, sound and think affects the energy and sensations in each cell of each organ of our body. Meditation is one of the easiest ways to control the body and lose weight.

Chapter 8

70 Weekly Positive Affirmations For Weight Loss

Positive affirmations are ground-breaking proclamations that we rehash to ourselves (either in our mind or so anyone can hear), and they are typically things that we need to occur. They are utilized to improve our internal reasoning and impact our conduct and the achievement we experience. Let's assume them normally with conviction and genuine conviction; your subliminal brain will, at that point, come to acknowledge them as genuine. This will strengthen your new positive mental self-portrait and accuse you up of positive vitality. When your psyche begins to think something is valid, your disposition, conduct, and thinking will change to realize a perpetual change. Positive confirmations can be adjusted to any objective you wish to accomplish, including getting more fit. Positive attestations are an extremely extraordinary device that you can use to assist you with shedding pounds. It very well may be trying under the most favorable circumstances when you are attempting to get more fit, particularly when you have melancholy, or you don't feel that great about yourself. Being overweight can cause a wide range of negative feelings that make it harder to remain spurred. Whatever you state to yourself greatly affects your circumstances and conditions. Truly the vast majority have no clue exactly how negative their idea designs are; have you ever gotten a brief look at your body in the mirror and felt your heart sink? Shouldn't something is said about when you state "I'm so fat and disturbing?".

These are both extremely normal instances of negative self-talk. Negative self-talk is a deadly inspiration critic just as being exceptionally terrible for your general confidence. Getting thinner takes persistence and duty, and in the event that you need to succeed long haul, you deserve to take the necessary steps to remain positive and persuaded. So what precisely are attestations? Basically, they are certain announcements composed or spoken in the current state that emphasizes the result or objective you need to accomplish. The initial step to utilizing positive confirmations is to consider what you need to accomplish, and afterward develop various articulations that mirror this objective as though it were going on the present moment. So, for instance, if getting more fit is your objective, you may state 'I effectively accomplish and keep up my optimal weight.' Or you may state 'I love and regard my body.'

Here are some metal instances of positive confirmations for weight reduction:

For women:

1. I effectively reach and keep up my optimal weight;
2. I love and care for my body;
3. I have the right to have a thin, healthy, alluring body;
4. I love to practice consistently
5. Everything I eat adds to my wellbeing and prosperity;
6. I eat just when I am ravenous;
7. I currently obviously observe myself at my optimal weight;
8. Losing weight falls into place without a hitch for me.
9. I am cheerfully accomplishing my weight reduction objectives.
10. I am getting in shape each day.
11. I love to practice normally.
12. I am eating foods that add to my wellbeing and prosperity.
13. I eat just when I am ravenous.
14. I now unmistakably observe myself at my optimal weight.
15. I love the flavor of sound nourishment.
16. I am in charge of the amount I eat.
17. I am getting a charge out of working out; it causes me to feel great.

18. I am turning out to be fitter and more grounded regularly through exercise.

19. I am effectively reaching and keep up my optimal weight

20. I love and care for my body.

21. I have the right to have a thin, healthy, appealing body.

22. I am growing increasingly good dieting propensities constantly.

23. I am getting slimmer consistently.

24. I look and feel extraordinary.

25. I take the necessary steps to be healthy.

26. I am joyfully re-imagined achievement.

27. I decide to work out.

28. I need to eat foods that cause me to look and to feel great.

29. I am liable for my wellbeing.

30. I love my body.

31. I am tolerant of making my better body.

32. I am joyfully practicing each morning when I wake up with the goal that I can arrive at the weight reduction that I have needed.

33. I am investing in my get-healthy plan by changing my dietary patterns from unfortunate to sound.

34. I am content with each part I do in my extraordinary exertion to get more fit.

35. Every day I am getting slimmer and more beneficial.

For Men:

36. I am building up a strong body.

37. I am building up a way of life of energetic wellbeing.

38. I am making a body that I like and appreciate.

39. My way of life eating changes is changing my body.

40. I am feeling extraordinary since I have lost more than 10 pounds in about a month and can hardly wait to meet my woman companion.

41. I have a level stomach.

42. I praise my own capacity to settle on decisions around nourishment.

43. I am cheerfully gauging 20 pounds less.

44. I am adoring strolling 3 to 4 times each week and do conditioning practices at any rate 3 times each week

45. I drink 8 glasses of water a day.

46. I eat foods grown from the ground day by day and eat, for the most part, chicken and fish.

47. I am learning and utilizing the psychological, passionate, and otherworldly abilities for progress. I will change!

48. I will make new contemplations about myself and my body.

49. I cherish and value my body.

50. It's energizing to find my special nourishment and exercise framework for weight reduction.

51. I am a weight reduction example of overcoming adversity.

52. I am charmed to be the perfect load for me.

53. It's simple for me to follow a solid nourishment plan.

54. I decided to grasp the musings of trust in my capacity to roll out positive improvements throughout my life.

55. It feels great to move my body. Exercise is enjoyable!

56. I utilize profound breathing to assist me with unwinding and handle the pressure.

57. I am a delightful individual.

58. I have the right to be at my optimal weight.

59. I am an adorable individual. I merit love. It is ok for me to shed pounds.

60. I am a solid nearness on the planet at my lower weight.

61. I discharge the need to scrutinize my body.

62. I acknowledge and make the most of my sexuality. It's OK to feel erotic.

63. My digestion is astounding.

64. I keep up my body with ideal wellbeing.

65. I can do this!

66. I am proud of my progress

67. I will continue to improve myself

68. I will continue to improve my body

69. I will put myself first

70. I believe in myself.

I advise you to focus on "5" self-affirmations per day. You must create your weekly plan!!!

Chapter 9

Remind: Love Your body

How do I love my body if there is no reason?

You look in the mirror and you are dissatisfied. Do you wish that your shape, your nose, your legs, your hair were like somebody else's? Why do we always compare ourselves? Why aren't we reconciled with our appearance? We have heard ad nauseam that we should love ourselves, despite our mistakes or flaws. This includes things related to our personality as well as our bodies. However, there are very few people who can accept and be content with themselves. It is not about not wanting to change. It is a commendable endeavor when one wants to achieve or retain their looks or care about looking more attractive.

At the same time, most people are much more critical, stricter with themselves than justified. They are continuously dissatisfied with themselves and don't see in the mirror what others see. Some girls feel a significant discomfort looking at each other, both because they don't like looking at each other in general, and because they don't like what they see. Where do these reactions come from?

What usually happens is that you don't look at yourself; you only see yourself with respect to that ideal of beauty that you have in your head. This is where dissatisfaction creeps in. It has to do with the theory of social confrontation. We compare ourselves with those we consider better than ourselves; self-esteem is negatively affected. We all have a model in the head, a term of comparison that we have built by looking at years of magazines, advertising, and movies with perfect Hollywood princesses. The mantra must become one and only one: there is no need for me to compare myself to that model because everybody is a unique, generous specimen, rich in the indications of what I am.

Life would be much simpler and happier if we could accept ourselves as we are. A lot of negative emotions would be released, we would have less stress, and more of the things that really matter come into view. The bottom line is, if we really need to change something, we can't do it until we make peace with the current state. This is a vicious circle.

The mind works, in effect, in a strange way. If we resist something, we get more of it.

After all, if we focus our attention on what is bad, we reinforce the bad. And what we pay the most attention to as we think about something will come true.

Everything that comes from you that relates to you is just yours: your feelings, your voice, your actions, your ears, your thighs, your hopes and fears. That's why you are unique. Be happy that you are different from anyone, that you look the way you do and that it is just you. Start to feel that it's your own body, not something separate that you need to live with.

Do you want your house to be just like anyone else's? Or do you love the little things that carry memories? Don't you love the atmosphere of your messy place after playing with your kids? And the plain curtain that you know you should replace, but which your mom sewed and looks so good? Or the piece of furniture that everyone says you should throw out, but you insist on it?

That's how you should feel about your body. You should understand that you don't need to compare it with anyone else's because it's impossible to compare unique things. In addition, who determines what beautiful and ugly mean? You should not compare your body to the celebrities' perfect-looking bodies. First, because they are adjusted with Photoshop and other programs, and they are not real. Second, because you are different, as is everybody.

You're not them. You should not only accept your body, but you should fall in love with it. Do you think like Bonnie? Do you think no one could love you because you have some extra weight? Then ask yourself the following questions. Could you fall in love with someone only if they are perfect looking? Would you really love someone because of their body? I'll go further.

Do we really love perfect looking people? I bet you prefer your imperfect companion instead of a perfect looking bodybuilder. You like the little faults of your wife, husband, kids, and friends because they belong to you too. We love imperfections better than perfections.

See? We don't measure people based on their weight. In addition, if you are happy with your body and your existence, it will also manifest in your radiance.

How should you love your body?

Sandra Díaz Ferrer, a researcher at the University of Granada, works with women who do not like their bodies and suffer from eating disorders. After years of observations, she published a study in the Journal of Behavior Therapy and Experimental Psychiatry, which reveals how looking at the mirror correctly can help in the treatment of bulimia nervosa. Her technique can be fundamental for all women dissatisfied with their image, or those who suffer from eating disorders. Imagine you have a fear of bugs that obsesses you. The psychologist might ask you to look closely at bugs until you get used to them, desensitizing yourself to the features that first terrified you. You can apply the same procedure to your body (Ferrer, 2015).

Here's an exercise that can help those who struggle to be happy about their own imperfections. You have to stand in front of a large mirror and look at yourself as if you were doing it for the first time in your life, like never before, taking time for yourself. It must be a constructive and very careful observation. No distractions, no work commitments, no notification to pull your attention. Only you and the mirror. In time you hate your body or any part of your body, stand in front of a mirror and look at yourself. Go from top to bottom and sort out your "mistakes". You will have to start looking at yourself from head to toe, objectively observing all the details, without comparisons or judgments.

- Remember what that part of your body has done for you. When did it help, when did it protect you, when did it do something physically useful for you? Say thank you for something that was of help to you. Learn to practice gratitude.

- Appreciate what you have and love your inner self. Don't let a scale or a size define your identity and skills. It is no use to criticize yourself fiercely when looking in the mirror.

Here are some ways to cultivate enormous gratitude in everyday life. When faced with a negative situation, do not be discouraged. Ask yourself instead what you can learn for the future and for reasons to feel grateful. Promise yourself not to be negative or not to criticize yourself for three days. If you make a mistake, forgive yourself and go on your way. This exercise will help you understand that negative thoughts are just a waste of energy. Every day, list the reasons why you feel grateful. The body is a miracle and you should celebrate all the gifts it has given you. Think about the goals you have passed, your relationships and the activities you love: it was your body that allowed you to do all this. Take note of it every day. Go to the other body part and do the same.

When you have reached your toes, return to your head again, to your face, and now, going downhill, just say to all your body parts, "I love you." Even if you feel a little stupid about it, don't stop. You see, you're going to have a completely different relationship with your appearance. And by the way, let's not forget, it's not a coincidence that it's called outer. What's inside is more important. But what's inside is visible outside. So use your inner self to love your outer, and you will be much calmer, happier, more satisfied and more confident.

Set the alarm and watch yourself for at least 40 minutes at a time. Doing so could change your life. Experts talk about the epidemic spread of body image disorder, a severe problem that leads us to see ourselves as inadequate every time we look at our body. According to research, 90.2% of women have an altered image of themselves and are not satisfied with their bodies, a fact that has a lot to do with how we look in the mirror. The mirror is your new weapon: from enemy to ally, but learning to use it in the right way (Ferrer, 2015).

Compliment yourself. You should consider yourself and treat yourself with the same kindness and the same admiration that you would reserve for those you love. You probably wouldn't direct the same criticisms you do to yourself, to another person. Don't hesitate to compliment yourself, don't be too hard on yourself and forgive yourself when you make a mistake. Get rid of the hatred you feel for yourself, replace it with greater understanding and appreciation. Look in the mirror and repeat: "I am attractive. I am sure of myself. I am fantastic!" Do it regularly and you'll begin to see yourself in a positive light. When you reach a goal, be proud. Look in the mirror and say, "Great job, I'm proud of myself."

Stay away from negativity. Avoid people who only talk badly about their bodies. You risk getting infected by their insecurities and dwelling on your faults. Life is too short and valuable to be consumed by hating yourself or looking for every little fault, especially when the perception you have of yourself tends to be much more critical than that of others. If a person starts to criticize their body, don't get involved in their negativity. Change the subject instead or leave. Wear comfortable clothes that reflect who you are. Everything you have in the wardrobe should enhance your body. Don't wear uncomfortable clothes just to impress others. Remember that those who accept themselves always look great. Wear clean, undamaged garments to dress the body the way you deserve. Buy matching briefs and bras, even though you are the only one to see them. You will remind your inner self that you are doing it exclusively for yourself.

Ask others what they love about you and what they consider your best qualities. This will help you develop yourself and remind you that your body has given you so much. You will probably be surprised to discover what others find beautiful about you, you have probably forgotten about them.

Surround yourself with people who love themselves. People absorb the attitudes and behaviors of the people around them. If your life is full of positive influences, you will also adopt them, and they will help you to love both your inner and outer. Look for optimistic people who work hard to achieve their goals and respect themselves.

Chapter 10

Hypnosis For Yoga Meditation

Losing weight - why yoga helps me

You may have wondered why most people who have practiced yoga for years seem to be less affected by weight issues. Should yoga help? The question must be answered with a clear yes. It can not be compared to a conventional diet. Rather, yoga to lose weight is a great factor that promote weight loss.

What is yoga?

Yoga is an Indian teaching based on a philosophy. It is primarily about the connection of meditation, the so-called asceticism and special physical exercises. Asceticism is a kind of exercise to repent. These are intended to stimulate the mind and body to overcome their burdens and desires.

In the yoga exercises, it is important that an increased body control is trained. The focus is on concentration and relaxation. It's about reconciling the mind and body.

Yoga is now a recognized sport. Until a few years ago, it was mostly attributed to pure meditation and referred to as so-called alibi sport. Today, it is accepted as a sport that demands much performance, discipline and agility from the performers.

Of course, it does not fall under endurance sports and has nothing in common with bodybuilding. Nevertheless, you can gain strength with regular exercise. Through a variety of movements and postures you also build your muscle system. However, it does not replace the abdominal leg butt workout from the gym.

Health basis for losing weight

The better you learn and practice yoga, the more you work on your mind and body. These reactions promote your health in many ways. That's the point that matters to you and your weight loss plans. You can use the exercises to create an optimal base that positively supports weight loss. You do not need a strict diet, although certain dietary rules should be followed.

There are countless stops in yoga. That does not mean you do not burn calories. No question, it does not strain as a competitive sport or jogging. Nevertheless, yoga creates the best conditions for you to lose weight in a healthy and above all natural way.

Why does yoga help you lose weight?

At first glance, it does not look like yoga exercises can help you lose weight. Superficially, that's the way it is. While a man weighing 75 kilograms would burn between 300 and 500 calories with one hour of swimming or jogging, with one hour of yoga he achieves a calorie burning of 150 calories. That's at least half of what you could do with more beneficial sports. Theoretically, you would be able to lose much less weight and less weight with yoga classes. But that's not the case, because the yoga exercises will help you lose weight in other ways.

STRESS REMOVAL

Yoga, as written in the outdated form, provides for mental relaxation through the meditative effect. It leads to inner peace. This reduces stress. Stress as it arises through the hectic everyday life, illnesses, worries and problems as well as overexertion, grief and emotional pain.

You need to know that stress, especially adrenaline, norepinephrine and cortisol are released from the body. These dominate strongly so that other processes are blocked or less available.

For example, the substances suppress the secretion of happiness hormones. These are directly involved in your fat burning. That means: less happiness hormones - decrease in fat burning. As a result, your fat metabolism slows down and you lose weight.

With the yoga exercises you solve the stress blocks and reboots the body processes, which are necessary for optimal fat burning. You can consequently lose more weight.

Stress reduction with yoga

Improved breathing technique

With the yoga exercises you will learn a special breathing technique. Calm and above all a deep, even breathing is a basic requirement for the right practice. There is a lot of importance to that.

In terms of weight loss you achieve a much better oxygen uptake. Especially overweight persons tend to shallow, fast breathing. Oxygen needs your body to make your organs function more optimally. Countless processes depend on the interplay of various organs and processes. With a good oxygen supply, the blood supply is favored. As a result, important nutrients can increasingly be transported to their destination. The organ functionality improves. In addition, your body recovers faster after physical and / or mental stress. This also influences a rapid reduction of stress.

Elutriation of pollutants and toxins

The yoga breathing technique ensures that more harmful carbon dioxide comes out of your body. It is a waste product of your metabolism caused by spent oxygen. If this remains due to a shallow breathing in your body, it can have a negative effect on your metabolism. This can have the following effects on your body, which make it difficult for you to lose weight or impossible:

Less excretion of excess fats

Limited fat burning function

Increased fat storage in the cells

Possible weight gain

Spiritual power

In yoga, you train discipline and perseverance. You strengthen your inner strength. These qualities help you to follow certain dietary rules until you reach your dream weight.

Furthermore, strengthened mental power leads to more well-being. You will be able to respond more calmly to unpleasant situations over time. This protects you from unnecessary stress and does not leave your inner balance unbalanced.

As a result, you reduce the chance of developing blockages that make losing weight difficult.

How does yoga work for losing weight?

The right yoga style

In addition to the reactions that are caused by yoga, one focus on losing weight due to Indian technology is calorie burning.

As already mentioned, yoga exercises usually result in less calories at the same time as swimming or cycling. There are different types of yoga, which are different exhausting for your body. Accordingly, the level of average calorie burning can vary widely. For a consistent and rapid weight loss you should choose a style of yoga, with which you can burn the most calories.

You can certainly see this as a sporting activity. In order to lower your weight, a regular "training" in the week is important - comparable to a fitness program for losing weight. Here you only lose weight if you pull it off and stay on it.

Increase fat burning

Because calorie consumption in yoga is relatively low for weight loss, your weight loss plan should also include plenty of exercise. You do not necessarily have to go to a gym.

It is enough if you use stairs instead of the elevator, replace short car rides with footpaths or cycling and often go for long walks. However, you can lose more weight if you dedicate yourself specifically to a fitness program or sport. Most calories you can lose in the following sports:

- Jogging - an average of 547 calories per hour

- Nordic Walking - an average of 447 calories per hour

- Swimming - an average of 436 calories per hour

- Cycling - an average of 412 calories per hour

- Skating - an average of 408 calories per hour

- Yoga and exercise - the combination makes it

Of course, to lose weight, you can focus only on exercise and exercise - without yoga exercises. But with the simultaneous exercises you additionally promote your stamina, build strength and above all: You activate many body processes, so that exercise / sports optimally affects your weight loss. Without yoga your body needs much longer until your metabolism gets going and improves your blood circulation.

In addition, yoga works long after. In other words, the benefits of losing weight with yoga last longer. The increased fat burning persists for days - until you stress your body and mind again and expose stress. In pure sports, you burn more calories only during exercise.

An increased fat burning you will be able to reach a maximum of 12 hours after the end of the training. Yoga gives you a perfect template so that exercise / sport can be even more effective.

As a result, they complement each other, letting you lose weight faster and more quickly. It is recommended to achieve a daily calorie consumption through yoga exercises and exercise / sports between 500 and 1000 calories.

nutrition

An important contribution to losing weight with yoga exercises is the right nutrition. It is not a calorie-conscious diet that you should resort to. Rather, it is a diet that is adapted to your type of energy.

High calorie food is of course not allowed. What you want to get rid of through the yoga exercises, you should not finally add to the body in a higher amount by eating. What your diet should look like, you will learn in the last sector. Information about the metabolism diet

Which yoga style to lose weight?

Hatha Yoga

The Hatha Yoga style is the most common form, as it is widely used in Europe and the United States. For you it is perfect for getting started. Here you will learn the basic rules of breathing and meditation exercises. Connected is the Hatha Yoga style with the so-called flow.

That's a fast movement. Yogis, as the users are called, speak here of dynamic, powerful outdoor dances that connect with the inner dance of breathing. That means nothing else than to harmonize movement and breathing.

In this way, energy is released, your concentration increased and your mobility promoted. This yoga style is less suitable for losing weight. You burn around 200 calories in one hour. This is a leisurely stroll.

Ashtanga yoga style

Much calmer than the Hatha Yoga style, it is with Ashtanga. Also here the focus is on the breathing exercise as well as the meditation. This type of yoga involves six different exercises. These build on each other in terms of difficulty with each other. In an hour you can burn about 300 calories.

This is roughly equivalent to a walk in a tight stride. Optimally, this yoga style is not suitable for losing weight. But it offers an alternative, for example, if your outdoor activity fails due to bad weather. Before you spend your time lazing on the couch, the Ashtanga Yoga style is at least a good alternative to doing nothing.

Power Yoga style

If you want it to work faster with losing weight, at least the Power Yoga style is required. This is roughly equivalent to that of Ashtanga Yoga - only more intense. Fast movements are required for the position changes. Heart rate and heart rate increase. In the yoga school, the course usually takes between 30 and 45 minutes. An optimal hour is one in which you can burn around 400 calories.

Vinyasa Yoga style

The style of Vinyasa requires a little stamina. The physical stress is comparable to a slow jog. It is not as intense as the formerly mentioned yoga styles. This is more about the asanas. Under it to understand the dormant stops. There is a smooth transition between the posture exercises.

During the holding positions, the muscles are tense at different parts of the body. This leads to the actual load and calorie consumption. This is an hour of these yoga exercises with an average of 450 calories.

Chapter 11

Hypnotic Gastric Band

What is the gastric band

A gastric band is a silicone device commonly used to treat obesity. The device is normally placed around the upper part of your stomach to help decrease the food that you're eating. On the upper part of the stomach, the band makes a relatively smaller pouch. It fills up quickly and slows your consumption rate. The band shows you whenever you make healthy food options, reduce appetite, and limit food intake and volume. However, it leaves you with a difficult option of bariatric surgery, which is a drastic step that carries risks and pains like any other gastrointestinal surgical operation. You should not experience these challenges when you can take a simple and less invasive approach to achieve the same results as in a surgical gastric band.

The gastric band for weight loss

So now you can relax and take this time to wind yourself down, and allow all those tensions to start flowing out and disappearing. So just bring to mind to remember that hypnosis is just self-hypnosis, that this is not something that someone will be able to do for you. Because hypnosis is simply a state of deep relaxation, which successfully helps you to bypasses your critical factors so that the suggestions that are beneficial to your true self will be readily received and accepted by your deeper unconscious mind.

After all, trance is an everyday natural calming experience, and you're entering into that experience easily and effortlessly. So start by asking yourself, if you've ever put yourself in a calm relaxing state before this moment, and if so, you can recall all those calm and relaxing states that you've formerly experienced, whether it's via your favorite hobby, an activity, a journey or a holiday.

The most important thing to realize is that you should bring to your mind, relaxation, and protective magical thinking practices each day in your waking state because you know that the practice imprints it in your mind. And as time goes by, it becomes easier for you to be able to gain the benefits of these experiences, which helps to promote self-acceptance.

Once they become permanently fixed into your mind, you will experience some positive changes in your life, and they will become active by helping you to create positive changes in your life that are for your benefit, and they will lead you forward towards a real realization of those changes. And as you speak directly to the deeper inner part of the self that controls your eating habits and weight, you will realize that you have been eating more food than the food that your body wants or needs. And also, you will realize that your mind controls your eating habits.

Now just seeing all those levers that you can adjust, you can then choose which one to use because you know that you have the power over your weight and your eating habits. And also you know what you're eating. The exact time and amount that you choose to eat are controlled in this place, which is the deeper part of your authentic self.

This part of the body is not your stomach or your appetite, but it controls your food, but it is your mind, and you get to ask that aspect of yourself beginning today, to develop new habits for yourself. And set new positive goals for yourself because you are laying a mental foundation for yourself, who is now a cheerful, attractive, positive, and authentic you. The great importance to this new you and your healthy, active, and attractive body is that you are eating less food, and you're happier.

The more you smile, and the more relaxed you are, the better you will look and the better you will feel. Also, you will be able to find satisfaction in eating less and pride yourself in knowing that each time you do so, you are rewarding your slimmer, healthier, and natural self. and you will know that the slimmer you are deep within you as you exercise, this new strength will grow. And as you eat healthily and sensibly, you will find yourself filling satisfied, and you will discover that the exercise makes it more reinforce and more natural towards your authentic identity.

Because it is like using and strengthening your muscles to become stronger and stronger, now eating sensibly becomes easier, easier, in a practical, and the positive way means that you are mentally asking your body the foods it needs, and then you are taking the time to listen to your own body quietly. And always check in with your body on the little food that your body needs from time to time, and you will be able to take time to integrate these ideas on a deeper level.

If you are listening to these and choosing to drift into a deeper sleep, you can just do so. Now just feeling good will allow your body to be able to drift down and go into a deeper and restful sleep. If you want to get up and continue with your activities, then you have to count from one to five, and when you reach five, you can then open your eyes and come back to the fully conscious reality.

And so on counting one, you should allow yourself to come back to full conscious reality with relaxation and ease. Then as you count two, come back slowly to your full conscious reality, and as you count three, take some nice deep relaxing breath. Moreover, as you count four, allow your eyes to open as if you've bathed them with fresh water, and now, as you count five, open your eyes completely and adjust yourself to your environment while getting ready to carry on with your day's activity.

What is the hypnotic gastric band?

If you would like to lose some weight without using surgery, then the hypnotic gastric band is the best tool for you. The hypnotic gastric band is the natural healthy eating tool that will help to control your appetite and your portion sizes. In this sense, hypnosis plays a significant role in helping you to lose weight without having to go through the risk that comes with surgery. It is a subconscious suggestion that you already have, a gastric band comes intending to influence the body to respond by creating a feeling of satiety. It is now available in a public domain that dieting does not help to solve lifestyle challenges that are needed for weight loss and management.

Temporary diet plans are not effective while maintaining continuous plans are difficult. Notably, these plans are going to deprive you of your favorite foods, since they're too restrictive. Deep down within you, you might have a problem with your body's weight since diets have not worked for you in the past. If you want to try something that will be able to provide a positive edge for you, then you should be able to control your cravings around food hypnotically. By reaching this point, you must try hypnosis, which has proven some results in aiding weight loss.

Benefits of hypnosis vs surgery

If you would like to lose weight without starvation or yo-yo dieting, then the hypnotic gastric band is the ultimate resort for you. This gastric band does not require surgery but only meditation and hypnosis. Therefore, it offers numerous benefits that make it the solution to rapid weight loss and craving healthy food.

It is pain-free: As opposed to the physical gastric band, the hypnotic gastric band does not require surgery which is associated with pain and routine follow-ups. Therefore, you do not need to worry about the risks you need to take as no physical operation will be done on your body. You only need to hypnotize and utilize the hypnosis to work on your body weight.

100% safe: As hypnosis is a non-invasive, non-surgical, and safe technique so is the hypnotic gastric band whose mechanism is initiated in your subconscious mind. Through the practice, there are no expected dangers and you learn about self-awareness and the course of your life.

Time-efficient: You do not need to wait for your vacation to acquire a hypnotic gastric band. The tool does not affect your schedule as hypnosis can be combined with most of your day to day activities. You do not need time off to adjust the band or report complications

No meal replacement or dieting: With the hypnotic gastric band, you do not need to stop eating your most enjoyable food. Instead, you develop a principle that makes you feel in control and enable you to lose weight consistently and naturally without dieting. You just exercise and unlock the power in you to make positive changes in life.

No complications: The fact that no surgery is performed in hypnotic gastric surgery puts away the worry about future complications. The ease in your mind plays a significant role in focusing your mind on the things that matter such as visualization and meditation. This way, you can put off negative thinking and live your life fearlessly and positively.

Helps discover your hidden potential: The use of hypnosis and meditation makes you learn about how to utilize the power of your mind in changing your perception and erasing negative thoughts. Similarly, you become capable of helping not only with weight loss but also with other psychological and social aspects such as confidence. In this case, hypnosis helps plant a subconscious suggestion in your mind making it stick and become a strong idea. Cost-Effective: Hypnotic gastric band does not snatch away your working time making you fully productive at your workplace with no deductions. In the same way, there are no costs in hypnosis and meditation as opposed to the physical gastric band. Positively living your life substantially adds to your savings.

Chapter 12

How Meditation Can Help You Acquire Healthy Eating Habits

Helps you manage your emotions

Part of being human means that you have feelings. At times you may feel more emotional than other times. Some of these emotions can lead us to emotional eating. You find that all you want to do is keep eating even when you are not hungry. This is an unhealthy eating habit that can cost result in weight gain or at times, lead to some diseases. Meditation allows you to take charge of your emotions. Instead of regularly being emotional, it allows one to find some solutions for the challenges that they are facing. As you focus your mind on analyzing them, you can easily come up with a possible solution.

Helps you avoid overeating

You might have been hungry the whole day, and all that you are looking forward to is laying your hands on a sumptuous meal. You find that you have invested your mind into thinking a lot about the food you want to consume. When you do that, your appetite increases. Once you get a meal, you end up overeating since your mind has already registered that you were really hungry. Regardless of the amount of food you consume, you have the urge to keep taking more. In the process, you end up overeating and regretting late. At times sweet food can make us overeat. It might be one of those good days where you are feeling energetic, and you get to cook a nice meal. You spend much of your time making the meal, and when it comes to eating it, you find yourself overeating since it is a delicious meal. Meditation allows you to know when you are full, and hence you get to understand that there is no need to keep adding more food. You get to eat the portion that you need, and you can save the rest for another day. In this case, it allows you to have self-control as you consume your food.

You find other ways to reduce stress

Stress eating is a major challenge among a variety of people. Life can get challenging, and you feel like you are under pressure. There are different challenges that we face. Some of them are beyond our control while others are manageable. You might have recently lost a loved one. The loss makes you feel stressed, and you may wonder why they had to go. An individual might be in a situation where they feel lonely, and this results in stress. On the other hand, you might have failed a test and you feel bad about the whole situation. You might probably be wondering if you will manage to graduate in the intended year or if you will have to stay longer at school. These are some of the situations that cause stress. When they occur, your solution might be eating. Anytime you feel sad or feel like crying; you end up looking for a meal to eat. In this process, you end up overeating, and the food consumed is not helpful to your body. Meditation allows you to come up with ways of handling such stressful situations and hence, one no longer needs to overeat.

It allows you to cope with eating disorders

Some individuals have chronic eating problems, such as bulimia and anorexia. Individuals with anorexia tend to deny themselves food. You find that they eat little portions of food in a day, which is lower than the amount of food their body needs. You find that some people struggling with weight gain tend to be anorexic. With weight gain, their self-esteem lowers, and they develop other complications. At times they may be uncomfortable around some individuals, and anytime they consume anything, all they want to do is throw up and release the food consumed. We also have some models struggling with anorexia. They want to be a certain shape, and hence they lower their food intake. They do not consume the required food portions, and it can have some harmful effects on their bodies. Bulimia refers to a condition whereby the individual consumes a lot of food, which is unnecessary. This is a challenge to petite individuals who want to add extra weight. You find that regardless of the amount of food that they consume, no big change occurs in their body. Meditation allows you to accept yourself as you are and hence, you do not need food to boost your self-esteem.

It improves focus

When your mind is in a calm state, your concentration level increases. You find that you become more focused on the task that you are undertaking, and you do it well. Eating requires some focus. For instance, while chewing, being focus can help you in proper chewing of food. In this case, all the food particles are well broken down. This makes certain processes such as digestion easier. When this occurs, the food consumed is well utilized in the body. In this case, all the food becomes beneficial, and none is wasted. It also makes the process of ingestion easier. The challenge of having excessive and unutilized foods in the body is managed. As a result, the problems that result from poor eating are also well taken care of. Focus is essential in all aspects of life. It improves our performance in the tasks that we are undertaking, and it ensures that we make the right choices. You might overlook the importance of focus when it comes to eating, but it plays a crucial role.

You eat only the required food portions

In some moments, greed causes us to eat more food than we require. Greed can result from seeing a good well-prepared meal and automatically desiring to have it. You might have eaten, and you were full, but since you came across a meal that looks delicious, you have the sudden urge to consume it. In that case, you will be eating not because you are hungry, but due to greed. To avoid some of those incidences, you need to have some self-control. When you have consumed the needed portion of food, you have to train your body not to need more. Even if you eat the extra portion, it has no use to your body since the body does not use it. It instead disposes it into waste since it does not add any value to it. At times your body will convert it into fat, and you end up gaining weight. On the other hand, some people misunderstand the concept of dieting and think that it means denying themselves food. You may find that an individual is skipping some meals just to lose weight. When you do this, you deny your body its needs, and it can result in further complications. To avoid this, ensure that you take the required amount of food.

It allows you to avoid impulse buying of food

Impulse buying of food is similar to impulse shopping. In impulse shopping, you find that you are walking around a shop with the intention of buying a specific item, but you end up buying items that you had not budgeted for. For instance, you might be walking to a supermarket to buy some groceries, but you end up buying a pair of shoes. You had no intention of getting the shoes, which means it is an added item to your budget. On the other hand, you might find yourself not using the item you bought because you did not need it in the first place. Such random purchases also occur with food. As you are walking along the streets, you may come across a fast food joint, and you automatically decide to get some fries. You initially did not have any plans to get them, but since you came across them, immediately, a need arises. Meditation allows you to make the right choices. You get to analyze the situation and decide on the best thing to do. In most cases, you will decide to forego making the impulse purchase

Helps in self-awareness

We have been created to function differently. Each individual has their own unique characteristics that set them apart from the others and make them who they are. Your way of thinking and doing things might be different for that of another person. At times you will get in an interview, and they tell you to describe yourself. What are the responses you would have to give? Most people freeze when asked this question because we are not aware of who we are. We barely take time to understand ourselves, and hence we know little about who we are. Meditation allows us to connect with our inner being. When you take some me time, you may decide to meditate about your life. This will involve asking yourself some important questions and your responses to the asked questions will tell a lot about the kind of person that you are. When it comes to acquiring healthy eating habits, self-awareness is necessary. You need to be well aware of the challenges that you will face while trying to adapt some of those eating habits. This allows you to easily focus and manage to successfully utilize the good eating habits.

Helps you follow your diet plan

Following a diet plan can be quite a challenging task. The first days can be challenging, especially if you have never tried it before. You may decide to have only one meal that is out of the diet, and you end up having more than just one meal. Instead of the one meal that you had promised yourself, you extend to a week, and before you know it, you are no longer following the diet plan. While dieting, you will need a lot of discipline that ensures you stay focused on your decisions. Despite the circumstances or the events around you, you always ensure that you stay focused on what you do. The biggest challenge with dieting is that you will always come across food. As you walk across different streets, you will come across food. You could also be sitting near an individual who is eating, and you feel tempted to get what they are eating. It takes a lot of discipline and self-control to ensure that you stick to your diet. Meditation allows you to acquire this kind of discipline and it ensures that you stay focused on your goals and plan.

Chapter 13

How to Overcome Mental Blocks to Lose Weight

What beliefs are holding onto your weight?

- I am inferior
- I am lacking
- I am inconsequential so I have to make myself big to be seen Losing weight is too difficult
- I will fail and put the weight all back on again
- I must be so awful and bad not to be able to control my eating
- I want to punish myself
- It is too hard to start dieting
- My weight is ancestral, and I can't change that
- My weight is genetic, and I can't change that
- I am not good enough/I am not enough
- I self-sabotage myself
- I am worthless
- I loathe myself

Healing negative beliefs

A pattern is a program that you have which is part of your personality. For example, in your personality could be the thoughts: I am not as good as other people

This means that you block your weight loss as you feel that the task is too daunting, and you will fail. New patterns can be easily installed using EFTTM.

A block is something that stops you moving forward and the biggest one of these is FEAR. The other one is being safe. If your subconscious feels that it is not safe it WILL NOT LET YOU DO IT. So, if your subconscious feels that losing weight is not safe, you WILL NOT LOSE WEIGHT!

Also, if you think you are worthless or you feel you do not deserve, this will cause you to self-sabotage.

Healing negative patterns and blocks

The best ways to heal negative patterns and blocks are:

- Emotional Freedom Technique
- Bach Flower Remedies
- Affirmations
- Meditation

What is self-sabotage?

The term, self-sabotage, describes our often-unconscious ability to stop ourselves being, doing or having; being the person we want to be, doing what we want to experience or achieve or having our goals and desires become reality.

Most of the time we are totally unaware that we are self-sabotaging as it happens on a subconscious level. However sometimes we are aware of that little voice in the back of our head that says, "you can't learn a language" or "don't be ridiculous you can't lose weight".

Our subconscious mind is a powerful tool and always thinks that it is acting in our best interest. Stopping us stepping into new territory, discouraging us from taking risks ensures that we don't get hurt, we are not humiliated, and we don't fail – that is why so many projects never get off the ground. Rather than playing to win, self-sabotage plays to avoid defeat.

The purpose of this aspect of the subconscious is self-protection and survival. It can even negatively affect your health if it thinks that this will protect you from greater risk. Layers of excess weight have long been recognized as protection and very often the subconscious will use weight gain to protect you from perceived dangers you might be exposed to as a slimmer person. For example, where someone has been abused as a child, the subconscious may add weight to make them unattractive (it thinks) so that the abuse is never repeated.

So, people may talk about self-sabotage in regard to their weight because they eat emotionally and put on weight. However, sometimes self-sabotage will affect your hormones and/or organs, causing weight gain in people who eat only a modest amount. Sometimes people can lose weight but always put it back on just another method of self-sabotage. Once the perceived need to protect through self-sabotage has been healed and released, our illnesses and weight may disappear.

My experience of self-sabotage

In my personal quest to lose the weight and water I had accumulated; I consulted a lady who specialized in 'muscle testing'. When we asked the question "Do I want to be slim", the clear reply was "no!" which took me totally by surprise. So then started the journey of discovery as to why my subconscious didn't want me to be slim.

Why was I self-sabotaging?

During the long seventeen years in which I slowly cleared and healed the reasons for my self- sabotage:

I had set up a self-punishment/self-destruct program because of what I had done in past lives

I had set up a protection around me (weight and water) because of the sexual abuse, date rape and male attention I had had – I didn't feel it was safe to be a woman

I had several past life issues with starving to death and didn't want to starve in this lifetime

I had several past life issues with dying of thirst, hence the excess water in this lifetime to ensure that it didn't happen again

I had a tremendous amount of other karma

I thought that if I became a therapist I could not trust myself not to hurt, or experiment on patients, as I had hurt them before in past lives and so I was only going to be a therapist when I was 'slim'

I was frightened to take herbs as I had seen so many people die from them in past lives

Because I had been persecuted in past lives for healing people, I thought I would be persecuted in this life as well

I was frightened of being powerful

I was frightened to do the work I was supposed to do

I was frightened that the volume would fail

Although I relate to my self-sabotage with weight and health there were many other areas of my life that affected.

I was always in debt and could never pay off my credit cards

I never got the job I deserved and was very often out of work

If I got a job, there would always be someone giving me a tough time (karmic payback!)

When I had any treatments, such as red vein treatment or plastic surgery, it would always go wrong

Believe it or not, my subconscious was creating a reality where all of the above occurred – the subconscious is that strong, believe me. Even when I had released the attachments, and got rid of the influence of my mother, my subconscious was still following their examples and as I strived to get better my subconscious really kicked in and made it worse.

So, my subconscious was actually affecting all my organs and making them work inefficiently so that I put on six stone and swelled up with water. This was because my subconscious knew I could lose weight and it decided this was the best plan of attack. That's why some people lose weight and then put it back on. The subconscious doesn't always realize what is happening to begin with, hence the weight loss. It then kicks in big time in survival mode and the weight goes back on. You would not lose six stone and then put it back on again – you might put back a stone and then get it off. People blame diets or losing it too quickly but, in fact, it is simply your subconscious sabotaging you.

Emotional and comfort eating

When you read magazine articles they always talk about emotional eating and weight gain. Some people do eat for emotional reasons and boredom. Some people do overeat and there are explanations for this. You need to identify your emotional eating triggers and use a technique such as EFTTM to eliminate them. However, if you want to eat try to wait for a 10-minute period breathing deeply and you should find that after that the need to eat has gone.

However, I know a lot of slim people who overeat and drink too much. They overeat for emotional reasons as well – slim people aren't perfect or without their own problems.

One of the reasons I wrote this piece is to show that overweight people do not eat emotionally any more than slim/normal people. How often are you on holiday and you watch people eat an enormous breakfast, followed by an enormous lunch and then three courses for dinner, plus booze, every day for two weeks? How often do you see a slim person eat a packet of biscuits or a bar of chocolate? ALL THE TIME!

You have to find the reasons why your subconscious doesn't want to lose weight and either release the reasons if these are past lives based or change your subconscious 'belief system' if they are more personality traits.

Removing the self-sabotage

When I was spending a huge amount of money with therapists and nothing worked, I did mention that I might be self-sabotaging myself. Most of them threw their hands up in horror and told me it was just an excuse to overeat (here we go again, I thought).

I read a lot about Emotional Freedom Technique (EFTTM) and in the very first paragraph, I read it mentioned self-sabotage. This was quite amazing. However, my self-sabotage was so deeply ingrained that for a long time EFTTM just made everything worse, as my subconscious tried to hold onto its control of me.

I, therefore, had to dig much deeper by clearing the attachments, past lives, and karma and then I could use EFTTM and my other techniques to change my subconscious perception and its belief system that "I did not deserve".

Psychological reversal

I thought I wanted to lose weight, but I actually didn't and my subconscious was stopping me. You need to find out all the reasons why and release and heal them one by one. For this, you use the EFTTM psychological reversal techniques.

How are you self-sabotaging because my experience would lead me to believe that you are?

Habit of self-sabotage

I had a spiritual reading session and was told that the self-punishment had been healed but that I still had the 'habit' and that needed to be healed and not recreated. As it would have never occurred to me that I still had the habit and was capable of recreating the habit at any time. Our body and subconscious sabotage us so much that it becomes automatic and then a habit. So even when the original stimuli are healed the habit remains. So, remember to test to see whether there is a habit and then heal accordingly (normally the same way you healed the original pattern). Make sure you don't recreate the habit by repeating affirmations and if you feel yourself slipping back into 'deserving the pattern' immediately cancel this feeling and ensure that you keep healing it.

Chapter 14

Deep Sleep Meditation For Weight Loss

What is deep sleep meditation?

One of the best ways to really become relaxed and find the peace needed for better sleep is through the use of a visualization technique. For this, you will want to ensure that you are in a completely relaxing and comfortable place. This reading will help you be more centered on the moment, alleviate anxiety, and wind down before bed.

Listen to it as you are falling asleep, whether it's at night or if you are simply taking a nap. Ensure the lighting is right and remove all other distractions that will keep you from becoming completely relaxed.

Meditation for a Full Night's Sleep

You are laying in a completely comfortable position right now. Your body is well-rested, and you are prepared to drift deeply into sleep. The deeper you sleep, the healthier you feel when you wake up.

Your eyes are closed, and the only thing that you are responsible for now is falling asleep. There isn't anything you should be worried about other than becoming well-rested. You are going to be able to do this through this guided meditation into another world.

It will be the transition between your waking life and a place where you are going to fall into a deep and heavy sleep. You are becoming more and more relaxed, ready to fall into a trance-like state where you can drift into healthy sleep.

Start by counting down slowly. Use your breathing in fives in order to help you become more and more asleep.

Breathe in for ten, nine, eight, seven, six, and out for five, four, three, two, and one. Repeat this once more. Breathe in for ten, nine, eight, seven, six, and out for five, four, three, two, and one.

You are now more and more relaxed, more and more prepared for a night of deep and heavy sleep. You are drifting away, faster and faster, deeper and deeper, closer and closer to a heavy sleep. You see nothing as you let your mind wander.

You are not fantasizing about anything. You are not worried about what has happened today, or even farther back in your past. You are not afraid of what might be there going forward.

You are not fearful of anything in the future that is causing you panic.

You are highly aware of this moment that everything will be OK. Nothing matters but your breathing and your relaxation. Everything in front of you is peaceful. You are filled with serenity and you exude calmness. You only think about what is happening in the present moment where you are becoming more and more at peace.

Your mind is blank. You see nothing but black. You are fading faster and faster, deeper and deeper, further and further. You are getting close to being completely relaxed, but right now, you are OK with sitting here peacefully.

You aren't rushing to sleep because you need to wind down before bed. You don't want to go to bed with anxious thoughts and have nightmares all night about the things that you are fearing. The only thing that you are concerning yourself with at this moment is getting nice and relaxed before it's time to start to sleep.

You see nothing in front of you other than a small white light. That light becomes a bit bigger and bigger. As it grows, you start to see that you are inside a vehicle. You are laying on your bed, everything around you is still there. Only, when you look up, you see that there is a large open window, with several computers and wheels out in front of you.

You realize that you are in a spaceship floating peacefully through the sky. It is on auto-pilot, and there is nothing that you have to worry about as you are floating up in this spaceship. You look out above you and see that the night sky is more gorgeous than you ever could have imagined.

All that surrounds you is nothing but beauty. Bright stars are twinkling against a black backdrop. You can make out some of the planets. They are all different than you would ever have imagined. Some are bright purple, others are blue. There are detailed swirls and stripes that you didn't know were there.

You relax and feel yourself floating up in this space. When you are here, everything seems so small. You still have problems back home on Earth, but they are so distant that they are almost not real. Some issues make you feel as though the world is ending, but you see now that the entire universe is still doing fine, no matter what might be happening in your life. You are not concerned with any issues right now.

You are soaking up all that is around you. You are so far separated from Earth, and it's crazy to think about just how much space is out there for you to explore. You are relaxed, looking around. There are shooting stars all in the distance. There are floating rocks passing by your ship. You are floating around, feeling dreamier and dreamier.

You are passing over Earth again, getting close to going back home. You are going to be sent right back into your room, falling more heavily with each breath you take back into sleep. You are getting closer and closer to drifting away.

You pass over the earth and look down to see all of the beauty that exists. The green and blue swirl together, white clouds above that make such an interesting pattern. Everything below looks like a painting. It does not look real.

You get closer and closer, floating so delicately in your small space ship. The ride is not bumpy. It is not bothering you.

You are floating over the city now. You see random lights flicker on. It doesn't look like a map anymore like when you are so high above.

You are looking down and seeing that gentle lights still flash here and there, but for the most part, the city is winding down. Everyone is drifting faster and faster to sleep. You are getting closer and closer to your home.

You see that everything is peaceful below you. The sun will rise again, and tomorrow will start. For now, the only thing that you can do is prepare and rest for what might be to come.

You are more and more relaxed now, drifting further and further into sleep.

You are still focused on your breathing, it is becoming slower and slower. You are close to drifting away to sleep now.

When we reach one, you will drift off deep into sleep.

Practical methods to sleep meditations

Although you might be tired, you may still struggle to actually fall asleep because you aren't able to become fully relaxed. Going to bed doesn't mean just jumping under the covers and closing your eyes. You will also want to ensure that you are keeping up with incorporating relaxation techniques into your bedtime routine so you can stay better focused on getting a complete rest, not one that is constantly disturbed by anxious thoughts.

The following meditation is good for anyone who is about to go to bed. You will want to include this for getting a night of deep sleep, or one that will last for several hours. Keep your eyes closed, and ensure the lighting is right so that there is nothing that will distract you from falling asleep. No lighting is best, but if you do prefer to have some sort of light on, ensure that it is soft yellow or purple/pink. Always choose small lights and nightlights instead of overhead lighting.

Other benefits of deep meditation

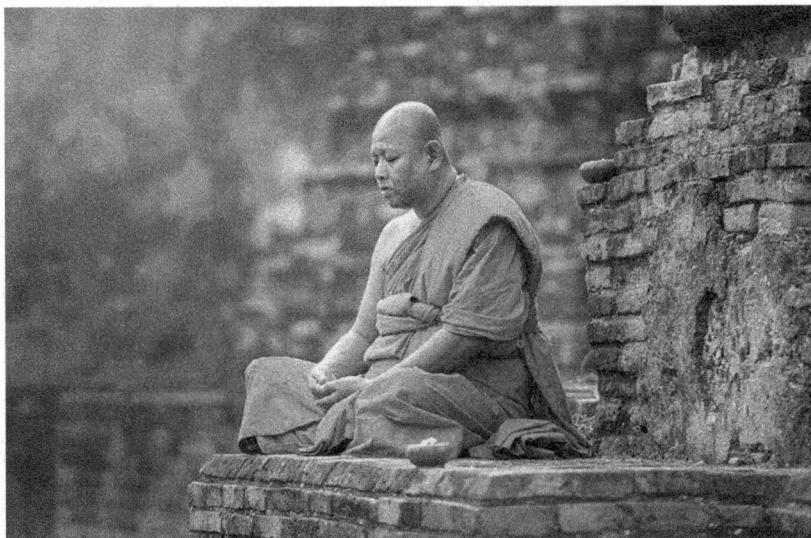

Meditation reduces stress

With meditation, you will feel calmer as well as have a stress-reducing impact on your body. With endless roles in life including work, children, and home activities, it is not surprising that you may be overwhelmed, which may contribute to increased stress. Unfortunately, these stressors affect your body by producing more cortisol, a stress hormone that affects the levels of sugar and insulin in the body. As a result, the hormone causes weight gain. Studies have revealed that meditation activates a relaxation response, regulating the nervous system and, in turn, lowering the cortisol levels.

With a few minutes of deep breathing and conscious relaxation, you will be able to obtain the cortisol-lowering benefits as well as your overall stress levels.

Meditation promotes a focus on intention

Often, meditation techniques involve focusing on specific goals or concepts. Meditating on cutting down weight streams your energy, thoughts, and intentions to a particular goal. In this case, you submit to the intentions by revealing your goals to the world, which makes both your conscious and subconscious mind to be aware of the goal that you want to lose some weight. The outspoken intention will stay with you for a long while, enabling you to achieve your weight loss goal both consciously and subconsciously, and dodging all possible distractions.

With meditation, you will learn conscious eating

With daily meditation, you will be able to boost your levels of mindfulness and awareness. This can allow you to live in the moment and always focus on what you are doing in the present. The process of meditation can help you gain an increased sense of awareness of actions and thoughts, thus helping you to think twice before you have taken an action. Rather than enabling your cravings to take over you, you will develop the power of controlling your mind, thus handling your cravings with greater intention and awareness. When you are ready to eat, your awareness will make it easier to recognize the textures and flavors of the food you are eating, instead of taking them for granted.

Meditation stabilizes mood hormones

Common daily stressors and activities can affect the way your system operates normally and may throw your hormones out of normal functioning. Apart from keeping your cortisol and adrenaline levels regulated, meditation goes further than this. The technique for relaxation releases both oxytocin and serotonin hormones, which boost your moods and ensure your hormones remain stable.

Meditation regulates sleep

Lack of sleep may hinder your weight loss progress. You see, by having a deep sleep, your cortisol levels will rise, which in turn will sabotage your progress in losing weight. Also, when you lack sleep, ghrelin, a hunger signal hormone, is also produced in plenty, thereby increasing your chances of eating more for weight gain. With meditation, you will be able to balance the circadian rhythms that promote quality sleep. Meditation increases the levels of melatonin, a hormone that also determines and controls when you sleep.

Chapter 15

How to Practice Mindfulness Eating and Shut down Negative Thoughts

The initial phase of "tuning" your own body for his own needs is usually not easy. "All of this is wonderful, doctor, but how is this to be implemented? I have work. I have children who need to be taken to classes, and I have absolutely no time to think about it! " To facilitate the process, I tried to formulate the most important rules. Usually, they write - rational nutrition, as if irrational - this is bad. And we will eat irrationally - as the body needs, but not the brain - and then it will answer us with gratitude, health, and harmony.

Another fundamental principle of intuitive nutrition: a varied food should be constantly available, should be nearby, at arm's length. Always. Compulsive eaters often have extremely little food at home, as they either diet or almost nothing can be eaten, or they are afraid of an overeating attack - and then it is better not to keep "dangerous" food at home. For an intuitive eater, it is important to have access to the widest possible variety of products so that at the right time, you can make the best choice that is in harmony with the needs of the body. Why is it important? Because having found the optimal combination at the moment, you will be satisfied with the minimum amount of food necessary for the current energy level of the body.

At home, at work, wherever there is an opportunity to make food supplies - make them. When you are hungry, you should have the maximum possible choice. What if hunger catches on the road or where food cannot be stored? Carry it with you.

If you went through all the prior steps correctly, then you gradually form the first stage of mastering intuitive nutrition. If characterized by despair, reduced self-esteem, and a feeling of inability to maintain another diet, go to the second stage of mindful eating - hyper consciousness at this stage, it is normal to pay increased attention to food and to be preoccupied with what, when, and how I eat, more than usual. You say - how is this different from dietary behavior? The fundamental difference is that dietary fixation on food consists of almost constant, anxiety, fears, and guilt. You are always afraid to break this or that rule, to eat the wrong thing, to make mistakes and be tormented, because you are surely mistaken, you are necessarily eating the wrong thing. You keep from doing anything all the time. In the second phase of intuitive nutrition, you do something completely different: constantly listen to yourself and ask questions: "Are you hungry? What do you want? This or that? Is it tasty to you? "And evaluate the level of your own satisfaction with this or that food. If this level is not high enough - this is not drama, not a disaster, not a violation of the rule. This is a training, valuable experience, and there is no personal guilt here - the food simply did not suit you. It happens.

At this stage, you begin to "reconcile with food," it ceases to be your constant enemy and rival. You do this by giving yourself permission to eat whatever you want. For many, this phase is experienced as frightening - a lot of people have never had such an experience in their life, so it is important to go through it at your own pace, comfortable for you, without haste.

At this stage, you will experiment a lot with food, trying it again, rediscovering the tastes forgotten due to many years of prohibitions. Paradoxically, it's a fact: allowing yourself to eat whatever you want, you may find that you don't like the products you dreamed of when they were banned. You may also find that it is difficult for you to stop when you are full, you continue to eat, having passed the saturation point. This is a normal process: restoration of contact with internal saturation signals follows after contact with hunger has been restored. It is important to follow this path step by step.

It is important to understand that hyper consciousness and the difficulties of managing eating behavior, even when you are already full, are not the final pattern that you seek to come to. This is a temporary stage in reconstructing your relationship with food as positive and free. Each of your food experiences ceases to be "right" or "wrong," each food becomes an instance in the collection of food experiences - not every instance of a true collector has the same value, which does not detract from the value of the collection as a whole.

This stage of mastering intuitive eating skills usually raises the most questions. Consider the most common of them.

Every Person Has "Priority Products"

This is the food that you choose most often in a situation where you need to have a bite, that food that is almost always "comfortable" for you (attention: this is about taste preferences, and not about the choice dictated by regular dietary considerations). Make a list of the food that you choose most often, and thoroughly stock up with the first five to six nominations in the list. Carry this food with you in a container for situations where hunger overtakes you on the road. This list is not permanent; it changes from time to time. The more accurately you listen to the signals of your own body, the more the list will change - you will proceed from the body's needs for certain substances without even realizing it.

"Hungry at the Wrong Time"

"I can't eat when I'm hungry, because I'm never hungry in the morning, then I run out to work. At work, I drink a couple of cups of coffee while I look through the accumulated mail, and so on until lunch. At lunch, I overeat, and until the evening, I remain with a feeling of heaviness from the stomach. "The task is to identify the moment when you are hungry accurately. If you don't feel like eating in the morning, hunger will catch you in 30–40 minutes. You will have to take food with you to be able to eat when you feel like it. Buy a large lunch box with compartments (even better for this purpose are boxes for sewing accessories, with many small compartments, each of which is closed with an individual lid). Put there what you like to eat in the morning - at least five different kinds of foods (yogurt, fruit, a little granola or cereal, small canapé sandwiches or cubes of cheese, ham, boiled chicken, small vegetables, nuts). It remains to get it at the moment when you are really hungry, and then I want to step back and talk about one strange cultural phenomenon that I have to observe while living at the junction of two different cultures.

The Dutch have the phenomenon of the "sacred sandwich" - whether it is a lecture at the university, an important high-level meeting, or a queue at the clinic - nothing will stop the Dutchman from getting a sandwich neatly packed in the morning and eating it decorously, without the slightest feeling of awkwardness. In the USA, according to my feelings, there is a rather powerful flow of awkwardness surrounding the "food taken from home." I can assume that this is somehow connected with the tradition of workers in factories and factories in the 1950s and taking lunch with them. And no matter how skillful the wife is in cooking, no matter how delicious the home-made food, it is rare that any of the Western office workers will decide to "go with them" as opposed to a "business lunch" in a cafe so that there are no unnecessary associations. Parents in childhood also teach children about "eating indecently on the street." The maximum that children are allowed is ice cream.

The only recommendation I can give is to take responsibility for your food and your hunger. You have the inalienable right to eat if you are hungry. And if you are hungry on the way to work, then you have every right to satisfy this hunger. This is much more important than what others will think or say. Yes, I know that the road to work is not always very comfortable and conducive to food. But as soon as you say to yourself: "It's better to tolerate" - you take a step back, running again and again in the wheel of satisfying other people's needs at the expense of your own.

Shut down Negative Thoughts and Feel Right

I can't eat in public (in transport, on the go...).

Many compulsive eaters feel they have no right to eat, not only on the road but in any public place, except for a safe place at home. This is especially true for overweight people. How can they feel free to eat if they are already fat, ugly, and unattractive? This sensation has a direct connection with the global feeling "not entitled," characteristic of people with impaired eating behavior: not entitled to demand, ask, expect. Not entitled to say no.

There is no better way to start working with your satisfying the needs of others at the expense of your own than there is at a time when you have a need for it. Having won back from yourself and those around you, there is a right when and what you want, you can hope that the feeling that you are entitled will begin to spread to other areas of life. Usually, at first, this is manifested by flashes of sudden, unusual for your anger and irritation where formerly you behaved modestly and unnoticed.

Do not be alarmed - this is how your autonomy is formed. The period of anger soon passes, giving way to the calm feeling "I have the right to do it," and this is a crucial stage not so much in the adjustment of nutrition as in the formation of a mature personality.

The theme of "give yourself the right" requires in-depth study, preferably in psychotherapy, if possible. You have no right to be hungry - what is it about in your personal past?

When working with these memories, with your resentment and anger, it is essential to continue to work with eating behavior, not to forget that these are two parallel, intensifying each other, processes. Being hungry, note that the fact that you are and going to eat doesn't affect at all and will not affect your relationship with other people. Perhaps this was in the past, but those times are past. Note also that it is unknown and entirely unimportant for other people whether you are eating now because you are hungry, or for other reasons. You deserve to notice your needs and meet them as they become available.

Chapter 16

Enhance Your Motivation

Your journey is going to start with your motivation level. Many things are possible, but it feels like almost nothing is when you are lacking motivation. Getting out of bed morning after morning, trying to find the strength to make it through the day can feel as hard as trying to climb a mountain on some days. Motivation can be found in many different things, but it will always come from our minds. What we're passionate about, the things that really matter, those are what motivates us to make it through the day.

The first thing you are going to want to do to motivate you is to change your attitude into a positive one. When we look at the world through a gray lens, we can easily see everything as terrible. When you hate one thing, that hate starts to grow and can spread into other parts of your life. We can't look at life through rose-colored glasses either, because we don't want to make ourselves ignorant to reality. We have to look at the world, at our life, head on, as it is in an objective way. When we can do this, it will be much easier to take on the new things that present themselves to you each and every day.

Give yourself time to prepare to be motivated too, not just time to start the weight loss. First, you have to get in the right mindset. Then, you can prepare for your meal plan and exercise regimen before starting. If you try to force yourself into it, you might sometimes make it even harder to get started.

As humans, we like to be independent. Not everyone is interested in being told what to do and we sometimes seek to be defiant in ways, even against ourselves. Sometimes in our heads, the things we're being told to do won't be our own ideas and can instead simply be the pressures of society, our peers, and our parents. Their voices can still get so deep in our heads that we will mistake them for our own and can easily get frustrated with what we're telling ourselves.

It can seem like an internal battle when you are trying to get motivated. There's the part of you that knows what you have to do, and then there's the voice that's telling you to just not do it. To just sit around and wait for tomorrow. Motivation is all about silencing that voice and building one of encouragement.

Don't allow any regret into your life or into the future. Regret can be such a wasted emotion. At the end of the day, it is not. There is a psychological purpose for regret. It causes us to look back on our mistakes and question our motives for doing certain things. Regret can teach us how to be better in the future. However, too much regret can lead to a lot of time wasted. There are some individuals that will be so regretful over certain decisions that it consumes their entire life. If you want to move forward and be motivated, not just about weight loss but with everything in your life, then you have to learn how to let go of regret. Feeling it in the first place isn't wrong, but don't entertain it anymore. Think of it like someone that you pass at the grocery store, someone that that you want to still is respectful towards even though you aren't very fond of him or her. Instead of talking to them and inviting them out to dinner, simply smile at them and keep walking. This is how we have to learn to process all feelings of regret, and emotions of guilt and shame as well. Simply let it passes, but do not allow it to stay past its welcome.

You are the person that you are right now because of the life that you've lived. It can be so easy to think, "Oh I should have done this," or "if only I had gone with the other option." However, if we hadn't made that one choice, then our lives would be incredibly different than what they are now. Each thing we've experienced, the decisions we've made and the thoughts that we've had, these are all like ingredients that go into what makes us who we are. When you can learn to love yourself and the person that you've become, then it will be easier to build that motivation because you'll let that guilt and regret losing.

Look at what motivates you right now, at this very second. What's the first thing that comes to mind? Maybe it is wanting to make a loved one proud or providing for your child. Perhaps your motivation is getting your bills paid or simply making your following meal. Whatever it is, this can tell you a lot about what drives you in this life. When you can become aware of all the motivating factors in your life, it will be a lot easier to use these images and ideas when you are struggling in certain situations. If nothing comes to mind at all, then it is time to do some soul searching. At the very least, wanting to make ourselves happy should be a motivator. Feeling good and looking better is all I need to motivate me on some days; however, others require a little more work.

Honestly, sometimes food was a motivator for me. I would tell myself that if I could avoid fast food all week and eat healthy Monday-Friday, that Saturday, I could go crazy. I told myself it didn't' matter if I wanted to drive myself through Taco Bell, Wendy's, and KFC all in one week. Whatever I decided for Saturday would be fine, as long as I stayed resilient against my cravings for Monday-Friday. If I was struggling on Wednesday and just wanted to skip the salad I brought to work and walk to the fast food joint across the street, I would remind myself that I could get it on Saturday. When I would diet in the past, I would think that I had to cut all bad food out for the time being. It would drive me crazy! Eventually, I realized that I had to give myself looser restrictions and reminding myself that it wouldn't be too long before I could have fast food again helped to keep me motivated throughout the week, rather than constantly thinking about the food that I wanted.

What would end up happening was that I felt so good about myself for eating healthy all week that I wouldn't want to ruin my streak so I would keep up the diet. I would get to Saturday and think to myself that I had done so well all week, why ruin it now? I might still occasionally go out to dinner with my family on the weekends and get something that isn't great for me, but then this was a reward. I realized that motivation would breed more motivation. The easier it was for me to get started with the things I want and stay focused on my goals, the more this strengthened my willpower. There are always going to be hard days, but I just remind myself that this is part of the process.

Your Dream Outfit

"Weight loss doesn't begin in the gym with a dumbbell; it starts in your head with a decision." – Toni Sorenson3

Some people will put pictures of their celebrity icons on their fridge, or maybe even their mirror, so that they see them when they wake up. You need motivation that will help you picture yourself in your future, not someone else's body and journey. If your main motivation is done by comparing yourself to others, then that's not going to be healthy in the long run. Instead, it might drive you to eat more because you are feeling bad about yourself, in more of a fragile state where you are going to decrease motivation levels. The thing about celebrity bodies is that if they aren't photoshopped, then they were still achieved through trick lighting and a team of makeup artists, as well as a personal trainer and shopper that gives them all the tools needed to lose weight. Most of us women are doing this on our own, so we have to stay realistic.

If you are 5 feet tall and you put a Victoria's Secret model on your fridge, that's not going to do you any good. We all have different bodies, and even if you were at your healthiest body weight, you might still not look anything near to the person that you are comparing your body to. Some of us are naturally curvier as well, while others might be stick-thin. You might have larger breasts and hips, or a bigger shoulder structure than many thinner models on the runway. We can't expect our bodies to look like theirs if the structure and height aren't the same, so using other people's pictures is never a good idea. It can just make you feel worse about yourself because you might get below your healthy weight and still not look like the other person, so you will still be disliking your body.

Right now, think of what your ultimate dream outfit would be. Whether it is a slim-fitting dress, or a cute crop-top and some butt - lifting high waist jeans, think of an outfit that you want to be able to look totally cute in. This is going to be your biggest motivator when you are getting started. You will be able to actually see yourself in this dress and be able to look at it with your own body, not just what someone else might look like. Be realistic with your sizing as well. Only go down a few sizes, somewhere that you would still feel good about yourself getting into. If you are a size 24 right now and you buy a size 0 dress, that's unrealistic. That could take years to get into, and there's a good chance that your body structure still wouldn't be able to slip into a 0. This is a small size and people that are a size 0 and have a healthy body weight are usually shorter, so be realistic. A size 16 dress would probably be a good place to start if you are currently at a 24. And if you are a size 16 now, then a size 10 would be good. Make sure you are aiming for something in between what your size is now, and what half of that size would be, give or take a number.

Chapter 17

Control Your Appetite And Your Food Portion Sizes

I t is safe to say that you are attempting to adhere to a solid eating regimen or weigh the boarding routine and thinking that it's difficult to control cravings for food?

Do you once in a while feel you are in one way or another subverting your endeavors?

The subject of craving the board can be a genuine bugbear when you set your focus on living all the more steadily. In the typical course of things, it's not something you need to give an idea to.

However, when you resolve to get thinner, or keep inside a solid BMI run, or even cut out nourishments that you realize aren't benefiting you in any way, you can out of nowhere locate that some physical marvels begin giving you sudden melancholy!

How needing to control yearning can trigger the craving

Maybe the information that you have in your mind that when you've completed this feast, there are X hours until the following one, pulls a prank on your stomach related framework and hunger.

Don't worry about it that, before you began your program, you were flawlessly well ready to get past X hours without uniquely considering nourishment. Presently that it's a 'fixed' time that you need to keep to, it appears to act as a trigger.

You may end up considering nourishment. It feels like you are as a rule so hard on yourself, denying yourself every one of those treats.

Seeing certain delectable treats, the scents floating from nourishment slow down, the menu hanging in an eatery window, also all that nourishment publicizing on TV, all appear to set your mouth watering and your stomach thundering. Never have X hours appeared to be so exceptionally long.

However, you truly would like to reach and keep up your solid living and eating objectives.

What would you be able to do?

A superior method to control hunger

Right off the bat, you can ensure that the eating regimen routine you are following is itself a sound and maintainable program, and not the sort of diet that drives your body into 'emergency survival' mode as a result of unseemly limitation.

Sadly, numerous well known 'prevailing fashion' consumes fewer calories have this impact and are best maintained a strategic distance from. Every single great eating routine will urge you to eat a sound, adjusted scope of protein, fiber, solid fats, and vegetables.

Besides, you can reinvent your appetite impulses.

You read that right. Even though yearning is an intuitive endurance reaction, how we handle it is, to a great extent, socially molded - that is, we've figured out how to be ravenous.

Furthermore, that implies you can get familiar with another approach to be ravenous. Also, the simplest, quickest, and the best approach to do that is with the assistance of hypnosis.

Hypnosis can re-teach your senses to control cravings for food

Control Hunger is a sound hypnosis session created by analysts with wide involvement with the field of weight reduction and the executives.

As you unwind and listen over and over to your session, incredible entrancing recommendations will be consumed by your oblivious personality. You'll rapidly begin to see that:

- your head is no longer pre-busy with nourishment

- your stomach and gut feel increasingly great and simple

- you never again feel overpowering cravings for food at 'non-supper' times

- you find that you normally neglect to try and consider nourishment between dinners

- you truly start to appreciate the more advantageous way you are living

The main 10 motivations to utilize weight reduction hypnotherapy

The following are ten top motivations to utilize weight loss hypnotherapy as an elective choice or on the side of a calorie-controlled eating regimen.

1. Hypnosis is a general sense that changes your attitude towards nourishment

Hypnosis treatment works by setting educative recommendations into the beneficiaries intuitive with the sole point of changing that individual's propensities. When utilizing this for weight reduction, your specialist will change how you center around nourishment, divide size, and your trigger focuses.

2. It makes you not have any desire to eat additional nourishment or treats

The mind molding the weight loss hypnotherapy gives permits you to progress away from eating or getting yourself the typical cakes, desserts, or chocolates that ruin your fair eating routine. Hypnotherapy works for weight reduction by re preparing the mind to imagine your optimal future weight and body shape. This at that point goes about as an impetus and in fabricated spark

3. Eating the correct nourishments gets automatic

The intensity of hypnotherapy will empower you to move in the direction of picking the correct nourishments forthright, not depending on prevailing fashion consumes fewer calories, gorging, or depending on sweet or remove nourishment suppers.

4. It inspires you to like eating less

Hypnotherapy will empower you to pick the correct part size for your suppers without the idea of being eager once more. Mistaken part estimates are probably the biggest supporter of weight gain.

5. Less nourishment fulfills you more

By decreasing your segment size and successfully your calorie admission, you will see a decrease in your weight. You will find that eating littler mixtures fulfills you as well as causes you to feel better about yourself as well.

6. It advances a general change in mentality that incorporates an inspiration for standard physical exercise

My very own considerable lot customer's right off the bat seek an adjustment in mentality towards nourishment. When they find that they have accomplished the psychological standpoint that a positive way to deal with nourishment can accomplish, a characteristic movement to sports or the exercise center before long pursues, and their certainty around their weight loss develops.

7. It replaces the old pattern of speculation, with another sure and positive "can do" frame of mind

Numerous individuals that attempt hypnotherapy do so uncertainly of what the outcomes will be. There are no assurances with hypnotherapy as much as there are no certifications with an eating regimen plan. Results will fluctuate from individual to individual.

Be that as it may, we reliably observe patients utilizing weight reduction hypnotherapy effectively, and they break their old pattern of reasoning and build up a "can do" frame of mind without being constrained into it.

8. It makes getting in shape simple by overhauling the subconscious personality

Weight loss hypnotherapy is intended to get your intuitive personality to have just settled on the choice to eat healthily, take the size of the right bits, the right groceries, and advances a nice sentiment when you do the entirety of that.

Reworking the subconscious personality is an amazing asset for weight loss and numerous different propensities treated by hypnotherapy.

9. Toning it down would be best turns into the new personality proverb

Weight reduction hypnotherapy empowers you to acknowledge that toning it down would be ideal. By this, we mean when you initially pick the size of the right part intellectually, however, see the plate as normally far littler than you are utilized to; it won't feel unique or clumsy or make a mentality of reasoning "that isn't sufficient."

10. The old completion your plate mindset is supplanted with I don't need to complete my plate; your craving is in a general sense brought down on a long term premise

Just as bit size, gorging is another type of self-misuse with regards to controlling our weight. Weight reduction hypnotherapy empowers the patient to progress away from an "I see, I eat" attitude to a progressively controlled method for eating that reacts to the body disclosing to you its full.

Who is weight loss hypnotherapy?

Weight loss Hypnotherapy is for everybody. Results aren't uniform and rely upon the individual in question. Determination, want, approach and need will have an influence on your result, yet in any case, you should give hypnosis genuine thought.

Would you like to get more fit?

A large number of individuals feel like you do well at this point. Christmas has been and gone, the merriments have brought a couple of additional pounds, and the drinking sessions appear to have proceeded from that point. However, where it counts, you know you're not so much content with what's happening, and you need to change. Perhaps abstains from food haven't worked for you up until this point, yet you're willing to take a stab at something that will give you the positive edge you have to control the yearnings you have around nourishment.

Chapter 18

Preparing Your Body For Your Hypnotic Gastric Band

T he physical gastric band requires a surgical procedure that involves reducing the size of your stomach pocket to accommodate less volume of food and as a result of the stretching of the walls of the stomach, send signals to the brain that you are filled and therefore need to stop eating any further.

The hypnotic gastric band also works in the same manner, although in this case the only surgical tools you will be needing are your mind and your body and the great part is, you can conduct the procedure yourself. The hypnotic gastric band also conditions your mind and body to restrict excess consumption of food after very modest meals. There are three specific differences between the surgical (physical), and hypnotic gastric bands:

- In using the hypnotic band, all necessary adjustments are done by the continued use of trance.

- There is absence of physical surgery and therefore you are exposed to no risks at all.

- When compared with the surgical gastric band, the hypnotic gastric band is a lot cheaper and easier to do.

How Hypnosis Improves Communication Between Stomach and Brain

How would you know when you have had enough to eat? Initially, you will begin to feel the weight and area of the food. When your stomach is full, the food presses against and extends the stomach well, and the nerve endings in the walls of the stomach respond. When these nerves are stimulated, they transfer a signal to the brain, and we get the feeling of satiety.

And, as the stomach fills up and food enters the digestive tract, PYY and GLP-1 is released and trigger a feeling of satiety in the brain that additionally prompts us to quit eating.

Sadly, when individuals always overeat, they become desensitized to both the nerve signals and the neuropeptide signaling system. During the initial installation trance, we use hypnotic and images to re-sensitize the brain to these signs. Your hypnotic band restores the full effect of these nervous and neuropeptide messages. With the benefits of hypnotic in view, we can recalibrate this system and increase your sensitivity to these signs, so you feel full and truly satisfied when you have eaten enough to fill that little pouch at the top of your stomach.

A hypnotic gastric band causes your body to carry on precisely as if you have carried out surgical operation. It contracts your stomach and adjusts the signals from your stomach to your brain, so you feel full rapidly. The hypnotic band use s a few uncommon attributes of hypnotic. As a matter of first importance, hypnotic permits us to talk to parts of the body and mind that are not under conscious control. Interestingly as it might appear, in a trance, we can really convince the body to carry on distinctively even though our conscious mind has no methods for coordinating that change.

Cybernetic Loop

Your brain and body are in constant correspondence in a cybernetic loop: they continually influence one another. As the mind unwinds in a trance, so too does the body. When the body unwinds, it feels good, and it sends that message to the brain, which thus feels healthier and unwinds much more. This procedure decreases stress and makes more energy accessible to the immune system of the body. It is essential to take note that the remedial effects of hypnotic don't require tricks or amnesia. For example, burns patients realize they have been burnt, so they don't need to deny the glaring evidence of how burnt parts of their bodies are. He essentially hypnotizes them and requests that they envision cool, comfortable sensations over the burnt area. That imaginative activity changes their body's response to the burns.

The enzymes that cause inflammation are not released, and accordingly, the burn doesn't advance to a more elevated level of damage, and there is reduced pain during the healing process.

By using hypnotic and imagery, a doctor can get his patients' bodies to do things that are totally outside their conscious control. Willpower won't make these sorts of changes, but the creative mind is more grounded than the will. By using hypnotic and imagery to talk to the conscious mind, we can have a physiological effect in as little as 20 minutes. In my work, I recently had another phenomenal idea of how hypnotic can accelerate the body's normal healing process. I worked with a soldier in the special forces who experienced extreme episodes of skin inflammation (eczema). He revealed to me that the quickest recuperation he had ever made from an eczema episode was six days. I realized that the way toward healing is a natural sequence of events carried out by various systems within the body, so I hypnotized him and, while in a trance requested that his conscious mind follow precisely the same process that it regularly uses to heal his eczema, however, to do everything quicker.

One and a half days after, the eczema was gone. With hypnotic, we can enormously enhance the effect of the mind. When we fit your hypnotic gastric band, we are using the very same strategy of hypnotic correspondence to the conscious mind. We communicate to the brain with distinctive imagery, and the brain alters your body's responses, changing your physical response to food so your stomach is constricted, and you feel truly full after only a few.

What Makes the Hypnotic Work So Well?

A few people think that it's difficult to accept that trance and imagery can have such an extreme and ground-breaking effect. Some doctors were at first distrustful and accepted that his patients more likely than not had fewer burns than was written in their medical records, because the cures he effected had all the earmarks of being close to marvelous. It took quite a long while, and numerous exceptional remedies before such work were generally understood and acknowledged.

Once in a while, the cynic and the patient are the same individuals. We need the results, but we battle to accept that it truly will work. At the conscious level, our minds are very much aware of the contrast between what we imagine and physical reality. In any case, another astounding hypnotic marvel shows that it doesn't make a difference what we accept at the conscious level since trance permits our mind to react to a reality that is independent of what we deliberately think. This phenomenon is classified as "trance logic."

Trance logic was first recognized 50 years ago by a renowned researcher of hypnotic named Dr. Martin Orne, who worked for a long time at the University of Pennsylvania. Dr. Orne directed various tests that demonstrated that in hypnotic, individuals could carry on as though two absolutely opposing facts were valid simultaneously. In one study, he hypnotized a few people so they couldn't see a seat he put directly before them. Then he requested that they walk straight ahead. The subjects all swerved around the seat.

Notwithstanding, when examined regarding the chair, they reported there was nothing there. They couldn't see the seat. Some of them even denied that they had swerved by any means. They accepted they were telling the truth when they said they couldn't see the seat, but at another level, their bodies realized it was there and moved to abstain from hitting it.

The test showed that hypnotic permits the mind to work at the same time on two separate levels, accepting two isolated, opposing things. It is possible to be hypnotized and have a hypnotic gastric band fitted but then to "know" with your conscious mind that you don't have surgical scars, and you don't have a physical gastric band embedded. Trance logic implies that a part of your mind can trust one thing, and another part can accept the direct opposite, and your mind and body can continue working, accepting that two unique things are valid. So, you will be capable to consciously realize that you have not paid a huge amount of dollars for a surgical process, but then at the deepest level of unconscious command, your body accepts that you have a gastric band and will act in like manner. Subsequently, your stomach is conditioned to signal "feeling full" to your brain after only a couple of mouthfuls. So, you feel satisfied, and you get to lose more weight.

Chapter 19

Techniques of Self-Hypnosis

There are numerous hypnotherapists in the world and there have been a lot of such professionals in the past. Many of new hypnotherapists have started using their own superb hypnotic techniques while most of them recommend the commonly used but effective techniques of self-hypnosis. Here I shall discuss the most commonly used techniques so that you can use the one most palatable to you. This combination is easier to follow at the beginner level as well as it is equally effective (in some cases more effective than using individual techniques). The combination that I have used is that of:

1. Progressive relaxation

2. Visualizations

3. Direct hypnotic suggestions.

This is the best possible combination for achieving your goals and the changes that you want in life. You can replace the progressive relaxation with the other methods shown below (which would bring you into the trance state). However, keep the visualizations and hypnotic suggestions as such and in the given sequence as they are the like the root and stem of the tree of self-hypnosis which you are going to plant in your mind's garden in order to grow juicy and desirable fruits out of them.

1. Eye Fixation

The main aim of this technique of self-hypnosis is to focus your mind. It also makes you simulate going to sleep and works well for hypnosis as well as self-hypnosis. This technique begins with raising your eyes upward and fixing your attention on a spot on the ceiling of your room and then maintaining focus on that spot. Then you have to give suggestions to yourself (you can record them if you are the beginner) that the muscles in your eyelids are growing so tired that these are feeling heavier and heavier with every passing second. The following suggestions would provide you the information that your eyelids are so heavy that all you want to do is let your eyelids close. Just rolling the eyes slightly upwards and then closing the eyelids is a signal to your subconscious mind that it's high time now to go to the sleep. However, you actually don't fall asleep but move into a state of trance.

2. Double Bind

This technique occurs when you provide a suggestion to yourself that actually possesses two choices within it. One of the two suggestions is much stronger than the other. People most often are likely to respond to the stronger suggestion.

Here are a couple of examples of the double bind technique:

I know my cook didn't like to fry and cook the chicken or to clean my room in my college days (I didn't have a servant for cleaning but paid the cook to do it). If I asked him to clean my room, he'd try to find a way to get out of cleaning the mess of my room (filled with tons of written paper sheets). If I ask him to fry the chicken properly before cooking it, again, he'd try and find a way to get out of the frying process. But, if instead, I offered him a choice, here's what used to happen. First, I ask would him, "Do you want to clean my room today or do you want to spend the whole time frying the chicken properly before cooking it?" He knew he had to make a choice. So, instead of focusing on some way to get out of doing whatever I've had asked him to do, he used to focus on which he'd rather do. Though he didn't like to do either one, he would prefer frying the chicken over doing my room. The double bind used to occur because he didn't want to do either, but he had to make a choice. And he would make the choice that is slightly more emotionally compelling choice for him. He used to have a much better attitude frying the chicken because he was able to get out of cleaning my room. Not only did I used to have a tasty fried and cooked chicken for dinner, but I would also have the privilege of cleaning my room myself as I and only I can keep the mess of papers in an organized fashion in my room (I hated when others clean/disperse the stuff in my room. Shhhh... Secret, don't tell my cook about it).

If you are an alcoholic, you are often conflicted about quitting drinking. There is a part of you that wants to continue drinking in heavy amounts because you enjoy drinking alcohol, yet there is a part of you that wants to quit because you know that is what is best for you health-wise in the long run. So, here is a double bind for you: "You can continue to drink in heavy amounts and poison your liver till you get liver failure and cancer and die a very ugly and painful death, or you can choose to be a non-alcoholic and live a healthy, happy and long life." Continue to present this suggestion of double bind type to an alcoholic (or to yourself if you are the one) during the hypnosis sessions. There's a very nice chance that the person will quit.

In fact you can use the double bind technique in almost any type of you daily problematic situations.

3. Eye Catalepsy

A bit of double bind is utilized in this technique. You have to shut your eyes so tight that you can't open them even if you want to. After you reinforce this suggestion several times in various ways, try to open your eyes even though these are shut so tight that opening them would be impossible. This causes your eyelids to quiver slightly (similar to the REM state). After this suggestion, give yourself another set of suggestions to relax even deeper. This is indeed a very effective technique used in self-hypnosis.

4. Staircase Technique

This technique is also quite famous in hypnosis scripts. This can be easily utilized in self-hypnosis procedures. One of the commonly used suggestions is to imagine oneself going down the stairs taking one step at a time. With each step downwards, you need to double your relaxation. The idea of going down into a much deeper state of mind is represented by the metaphor "going down". This is an effective way of deepening your state of trance.

5. Metaphors

It is quite common to use metaphors in self-hypnosis scripts. You can use them in the form of phrases, complex words, or even stories.

You could remain calm and detached and relaxed and simply observe the thoughts that metaphors present to you and see them as they really are. Metaphors allow your mind to make the relevant associations you need to make in order to solve your specific problems.

Metaphors are effective methods that land you up into self-hypnosis as the subconscious mind works best with imagery and symbols. The visual metaphors and symbols help you to effectively get a suggestion or a message across to your subconscious mind which gives you a good chance to make the suitable change you are seeking to make.

6. Progressive Relaxation

This is the most common and one of the most effective techniques used in self-hypnosis. The purpose of progressive relaxation is to help your mind to focus and your body to relax. This technique was first developed by Dr. Edmund Jacobson in the first part of the 20th century. He claimed that a muscle is relaxed effectively by first tensing it for a few seconds and after that, releasing it. It is this tensing and releasing different muscle groups throughout the body that produces a state of relaxation.

You need to relax the different areas of your body, with one area at a time, until your body feels completely relaxed. The attentiveness which is required by you helps you to focus your mind to the exclusion of everything else.

7. Conversational Hypnosis

Conversational hypnosis is said to have evolved out of the Ericksonian hypnosis, which is a branch of hypnosis named after Milton Erickson. This includes the use of double binds, indirect suggestion and confusion techniques. The formula for conversational hypnosis: rapport, confusion, and suggestion. And here's one such illustrated example.

When you are talking to yourself during hypnosis, and you already have a complaint/problem regarding enough workload at your office or overburden of studies at college, you need to first establish rapport and trust with the inner critic that lays insides you and holds you back. You can do this simply by agreeing with your inner critic. "That's so bad. Sounds like I have a lot of work to do there." Now, you have established rapport.

Now, you need to do a double bind by giving such a suggestion to your inner critic that has two choices within it. In this case, your inner critic will respond to the stronger part of your suggestion. "Even though I have a lot of work to do there, I never know when (small pause) I am going to feel better." This is the simplest form of a double bind. Now, your inner self is presented with two contrasting situations of feeling overloaded with work and feeling better. The phrase "I am going to feel better" is stronger because your inner self would certainly like to feel better. So your mind shifts from thinking about your feeling of being overloaded and exhausted with work to the likelihood of feeling better.

Chapter 20

Why Do We Struggle With Weight?

For anyone who has ever struggled with weight, life can seem like an uphill battle. In fact, it can be downright devastating to see how difficult it can be to turn things around and shed some weight.

The fact of the matter is that losing weight doesn't have to be an uphill battle. Most of this requires you to better understand why this struggle happens and what you can do to help give yourself a fighting chance.

While there may be physiological factors affecting your ability to keep unwanted pounds off, there are also a host of psychological, emotional and even spiritual causes that may be affecting your overall body's ability to help you lose weight and reach your ideal weight levels.

That is why this part is about focusing on those "hidden" causes, the kinds that go beyond the obvious aspects which are widely conversed in the mainstream media and by everyday folks. We are going to be talking about how you can look inward to see how, and where, things may need to change so that you can begin to turn things around and make a positive impact in your life.

The obvious culprits

The obvious culprits that are holding you back are diet, a lack of exercise and a combination of both.

First off, your diet plays a key role in your overall health and wellbeing. When it comes to weight management, your diet has everything to do with your ability to stay in shape and ward of unwanted weight.

When it comes to diet, we are not talking about keto, vegan, or Atkins; we are talking about the usual foods which you consume and the amounts that you have of each one. This is why diet is one of the obvious culprits. If you have a diet that is high in fat, high in sodium and high in sugar, you can rest assured that your body will end up gaining weight at a rapid rate.

When you consume high amounts of sugar, carbs and fats, your body transforms them into glucose which is then stored in the body as fat. Of course, a proportion of the glucose produced by your body is used up as energy. However, if you consume far more than you actually need, your body isn't going to get rid of it; your body is going to hold on to it and make sure that it is stored for a rainy day.

If you are asking yourself why the body does that, the answer is simple. Over thousands of years of evolution, humankind has struggled to have enough to eat. It hasn't been till about the last two hundred years that most societies have abundant amounts of food. This has enabled our generations to eat three meals a day... and a little more. Given the fact that our early ancestors would go days without eating, evolution has programmed the human body to store up as much fat as possible. If the body were programmed otherwise, it would have some sort of mechanism that would either shut off hunger and use up the fat that has been stored up or signal the body the get rid of excess fat somehow.

But, we're not there yet. Perhaps at some point in the future, the body will evolve such response. Until that happens, we need to roll with the punches and understand why we gain weight the way that we do.

Here is another important aspect to consider: sweet and salty foods, the kind that we love so dearly, trigger "happy hormones" in the brain, namely dopamine. Dopamine is a hormone that is released by the body when it "feels good". And food is one of the best ways to trigger it. This is why you somehow feel better after eating your favorite meals. It also explains the reason why we resort to food when we are not feeling well. This is called "comfort food" and it is one of the most popular coping mechanisms employed by folks around the world.

This rush of dopamine causes a person to become addicted to food. As with any addiction, there comes a time when you need to get more and more of that same substances to meet your body's requirements.

It's exactly the same as happens with a drug addict or alcoholic. They need to consume more and more of the substance they are addicted to in order to get the same rush. In a way, the body develops a resistance to the "happy hormones" released when eating yummy food. Therefore, you need an ever-increasing amount of these hormones in order for you to get your fix.

As a corollary to diet, a lack of regular exercise can do a number on your ability to lose weight and maintain a healthy balance. What regular exercise does is increase your body's overall caloric requirement. As such, your metabolism needs to convert fat at higher rates in order to keep up with your body's energy demands.

On paper, this is a rather straightforward process. Through the process of cellular respiration, the body converts glucose (or fat back into glucose) and combines it with oxygen to produce energy. This process makes it possible for the body to transform its caloric intake into amounts of energy which can be used to fuel the body's movements.

As the body's energetic requirements increase, that is, as your exercise regimen gets more and more intense, you will find that you will need increased amounts of both oxygen and glucose. This is one of the reasons why you feel hungrier when you ramp up your workouts.

However, an increased caloric intake isn't just about consuming more and more calories for the sake of consuming more and more calories; you need to consume an equal amount of proteins, carbs, fats and vitamins in order to for your body to build the necessary elements that will build muscle, foster movement and provide proper oxygenation in the blood.

Moreover, nutrients are required for the body to recover. One of the byproducts of exercise is called "lactic acid". Lactic acid builds up in the muscles as they get more and more tired. Lactic acid signals the body that it is time to stop working out or risk injury if you continue. Without lactic acid, your body would have no way of knowing when your muscles have overextended their capacity.

After you have completed your workout, the body needs to get rid of the lactic acid build up. So, if you don't have enough of the right minerals in your body, for example potassium, your muscles will ache for days until your body is finally able to get rid of the lactic acid buildup. This example goes to show how proper nutrition is needed to help the body get moving and also recover once it is done exercising.

As a result, a lack of exercise reconfigures your body's metabolism to work at a slower pace. What that means is that you need to consume less calories to fuel your body's lack of exercise. So, if you end up consuming more than you actually need, your body will just put it away for a rainy day. Plain and simple.

The sneaky culprits

The sneaky culprits are the ones that aren't quite so overt in causing you to gain weight or have trouble shedding pounds. These culprits hide beneath the surface but are very effective when it comes to keeping you overweight. The first culprit we are going to be looking at is called "stress".

Stress is a very powerful force. From an evolutionary perspective, it exists as a means of fueling the flight-or-fight response. Stress is the human response to danger. When a person senses danger, the body begins to secrete a hormone called "cortisol". When cortisol begins running through the body, it signals the entire system to prep for a potential showdown. Depending on the situation, it might be best to hightail it out and life to fight another day.

Regardless of the outcome, the main point is to ensure survival. This evolutionary trait is what has helped preserve the human species throughout thousands of years. In modern life though, stress plays a very different role.

In our modern way of life, stress isn't so much a response to life and death situations (though it can certainly be), rather it is the response to situations that are deemed as "conflictive" by the mind. This could be a confrontation with a co-worker, bumper to bumper traffic, or any other type of situation in which a person feels vulnerable in some way.

Over the course of our lives, we are subjected to countless interactions in which we must deal with stress. In general terms, the feelings of alertness subside when the perceived threat is gone. However, when a person is exposed to prolonged periods of stress, any number of changes can happen.

One such change is overexposure to cortisol. When there is too much cortisol in the body, the body's overall response is to hoard calories, increase the production of other hormones such as adrenaline and kick up the immune system's function.

This response by the body is akin to the panic response that the body would assume when faced with prolonged periods of hunger or fasting. As a result, the body needs to go into survival mode. Please bear in mind that the body has no clue if it is being chased by a bear, dealing with a natural disaster or just having a bad day at the office. Regardless of the circumstances, the body is faced with the need to ensure its survival. So, anything that it eats, goes straight to fat stores.

Moreover, a person's stressful situation makes them search for comfort and solace. There are various means of achieving this. Food is one of them. So is alcohol consumption. These two types of comforts lead to high consumption of calories. Again, when the body is in high gear, it will store as many calories and keep them in reserve.

This what makes you gain weight when you are really, really stressed out.

Now, suppose you go on a low-carb crash diet. Your body is already under duress from the amount of stress it is under. On top of that, you choose to take away its usual caloric intake. What do you think will be the body's response? A further deepening of its panic mode. This is the main reason why crash diets only partially work.

Another of the sneaky culprits is sleep deprivation. In short, sleep deprivation is sleeping less than the recommended 8 hours that all adults should sleep. In the case of children, the recommended amount of sleep can be anywhere from 8 to 12 hours, depending on their age.

Granted, some adults can function perfectly well with less than 8 hours' sleep. There are folks who can function perfectly well with 6 hours' sleep while there are folks who are shattered when they don't get 8 or even more hours' sleep. This is different for everyone as each individual is different in this regard.

That being said, sleep deprivation can trigger massive amounts of cortisol. This, fueled by ongoing exposure to stress, leads the body to further deepening its panic mode.

Chapter 21

Particular Meditations
to Lose Weight

Remember that you will attain the right weight according to your body, and you should avoid putting your concentration on things like what the fashion industry tries to portray or advertising agencies that do not give the correct impression when it comes to weight. A healthy body is what you need, and you must avoid things views that may distract you from achieving your weight goals and living the life you need. Something you must put into consideration is your diet as you do these meditation exercises. The diet you take should entirely be determined by what body needs and not factors like your emotional state and the wrong eating habits you have cultivated before. As you continue reading this, you will eventually understand the relationship between these meditations and diet.

What you should do is read all the meditations in this stage then do each of them at least three or four times before you can choose the particular one that, you will concentrate on. Before you can evaluate and know what modifications you should do, try to do them four to eight weeks. You need to include these in your program so that they can be beneficial to you eventually.

Thousand Lotus Petal

This meditation called the Thousand Petal Lotus, is concerned with dieting, and it is mostly practiced in the eastern world. Meditation enables you to discover that everything in nature is connected. This exercise has with time been adapted to do away with several problems like how we are using it here to maintain a healthy weight. During this exercise, you examine 'inner self' but not focusing merely on an object like crystal. To start this meditation, you should first choose a word and make it be at the lotus center. For example, you can choose a world like 'fat' or 'hungry.' When you get yourself comfortable, you regard it, and soon you will start having a connection with it. If you choose the word 'hungry,' the association could be 'full.' This means that there are three things to consider. You now have the connection between the two words and the words. You need to understand why you choose the two words and their relationship. When you go back to 'hungry,' regard it and wait to see what you would associate after.

Your following association could be 'starving.' Think of the relationship between the two for a few seconds and try to understand the connection. Now go back to your word again and see what your following association would be. What if the association you discovered afterward was 'roof?' When you look at the three things, you may not get the connection. Even if you do not understand what connection there is, go to the center word and wait for a few seconds. You should not take these associations to be free, whereby you move from one association to another. The concept is that you should always go to the original word of your choice even if you do not understand their connection with the association. These associations may attract you, but even when they seem to come from the deep insights of your body ensure that you stick to the discipline of performing them, and you can probably evaluate these feelings when you are finished with the meditation, not during the meditation periods. When you are not disciplined enough when meditating, you will discover that there are a lot of techniques brought about by these associations to resist what you are doing. The resistance techniques are not so helpful to you because they will turn out to be with no substance. The best and most fascinating techniques come from following your meditations seriously and staying with the discipline. When you follow, the meditations without being distracted by these associations that come along, you will get real insights with substance. Note that you will discover these insights after you have finished a number of sessions, and you may not see results immediately. This is why you should be patient and wait until your real results can come. These results may also not come the specific moment you are performing the meditations.

In most cases, you encounter this form of resistance whereby you feel that when you leave the meditation exercises and follow an association that has come up or follows an association technique that is free, you may discover something that is helpful to you and learn more things about yourself. The resistance also seems to inform you that you will learn many insightful things about the universe. These are the feelings that you note at once as you perform the meditation exercises because they will lead you away from your discipline, and you may not achieve the desired outcomes of the meditations unless you commit yourself and learn how you can resist them. But the truth is that it is not easy to learn this unless you gain insights from experience. Therefore, the best thing to do is to ensure that you try to be disciplined and when you find that you have been led to join this smile to yourself because this is the nature of human beings and get back to your track.

Blue Water Technique

In the second mediation, an individual can learn how to deal with various kinds of pains. To start with, this meditation, you first ensure that you are in a comfortable position then get to listen to your body with the goal of knowing the part of your body where you can feel hunger. Try to understand your body with all your consciousness and know where hunger is located.

The hunger may be in your stomach or may also be in a different part of your body. Take your time and try to think where the source of the hunger could be. You need to explore all parts of your body, and if you are in a comfortable position and also relaxed, you will be able to ask yourself, "Is this part of my body where I feel hunger?"

After you have located the part, you can now see its dimensions with care. For example, some of the things you could note are; the shape of the part of the body, how deep and how long it is. Visualize that it is a shape that ends, sides, top, and bottom. Now think of this shape being filled with blue water without caring about the source of the water. Use your mind to let the blue water fill the empty space slowly. After that, now think of the water draining out slowly through the empty walls space and through the skin and to the floor, after which it leaves completely, and there is no sign of spot, wetness, or trace is left behind. Imagine the space being filled with the blue water again, repeat the same process, and do this severally.

When doing this exercise for the first time, it may take you time, like about an hour, because, for the first time, you will be searching your body to discover the part where hunger is located. After you have defined the part, you can now speed up the meditation so that the filling and draining happen three to four times, and this can take up to fifteen minutes. If you find yourself doing this in less than fifteen minutes, it means that you are too fast, and you need to slow down. While doing this exercise, you will also encounter resistance, and the most common would be this happening so fast, while at this time there is no concentration in the brain as it is going in different ways with what you are doing. You need to keep yourself concentrated and ensure that you can control yourself and be in control of the pace at which you perform the exercise. When you through do not forget that you need to have a moment where you do not have any agenda to evaluate your feeling and get the answer.

Apart from the meditation program, you select the weight loss goal. There is also another one, which should be done by everyone. If you are the kind of person who finds this particular one being distasteful, then you may decide to skip, but if you are okay with it, you can proceed first before starting one of your choices for weight loss. Note that you do not perform this at the time of your meditation exercise, but you should perform it either before you take your meals or after. You can choose one meal in a day when you will be doing this exercise but when you find that your lifestyle is too busy to perform it frequently choose a day when you can manage and a meal you are sure you can perform. This form of meditation has existed for many years, it is found in both western and eastern meditation schools. You will not need to use an object of your choice as you did in the earlier part, but you will be using the food that you are taking at a particular moment.

You can do this when you are alone or with someone who is also performing the same because it is when it can work well and ensure that you eat the meal in silence. After you put the food on the table, sit down to it. But when you are eating this time, do not do it like you are used to. Many people eat while their minds are roaming from one point to another. You may also be used to eating while being distracted, like watching television or doing something else like reading a novel. This time ensure that you are concentrating on the activity of eating your meal. Make sure that you are being conscious about eating exercise and feel what is taking place in your mouth. Also, ensure that you are aware of what is happening in the mouth and try to understand your feelings and the taste of the food that you are eating.

Chapter 22

Background Information Required for Weight Loss

Understand Your Habits

You may find yourself developing some habits without knowing. The same applies to create excellent health practice. Your daily practices and choices explain your current conditions. Stop complaining; do focus on your habits a remember your preferences will define who you will be. Albert Einstein goes on to say, "we cannot solve our problems with the same thinking we used when we created them." Step out of your bubble a given structure for the desired outcome. Really the hardest part is starting and you've already done that, and it will only get more accessible and more natural the more you participate and the more you take an active role in this journey. Consider habits development as elaborated in the story of a Miller and a camel on a winter day. It was freezing outside, and while the miller was asleep, he was awakened by some noise on the door. Upon opening his eyes, he heard the voice of a camel complaining that it was cold outside and was requesting to warm his nose inside. Miller agreed that he was only to insert the nozzle. The camel put his forehead then the neck, then other parts of the body than the whole body bit by bit until he started destroying things inside. He started walking in the house, stumbling on anything on its way. When the miller ordered the camel to move out, the came boasted that he was comfortable inside and would not leave. The camel went further to tell the miller that he could leave at his pleasure. The same goes for a habit that comes knocking about and taking over. Maybe you started out smoking your first cigarette, thinking it was disgusting, and then years go by, and you have a nasty habit. Well, bad habits can sneak in, but the same philosophy can apply to ethical practices. Just take it bit by bit and step by step, and before you know it, you have healthy habits in your life. There are so many challenges to healthy eating. You have to be willing to have an open mind and reset your thinking on food.

It is cheaper to develop new habits; effort is the primary requirement, but not that much. When you have trained yourself new patterns, train on it every day for some time, after which it will be automatic. We can relate that situation to a football club Coash who engages in various rigorous training with his players while awaiting the actual match. They practice new skills and moves. When match day arrives, the coach sits with the substitutes while watching the players playing from the line. Players play as per the learned skills and moves. Apply the required effort to actualize your goal.

While storying with your workmates, tell them how you drink 3 to for four glasses of water every day, the same as tea. That looks strict. In heart, you know how your consumption of water and team is reduced while at home. This is self-discipline. Self-discipline calls for the establishment of strong foundations. Efforts adopted is less.

Apply Core solutions

Recognize and face the challenges of healthy eating and develop new habits. Like a logger trying to clear a log, identify the critical side of each situation. The well-experienced logger will try to identify essential joints by climbing up then do the clearing. A less experienced logger would start by the edge. Both methods produce expected results, but one way saves more time and uses less energy than the other. All our problems have strategic points. How about when we identify critical logs to healthy eating and offer some solutions. First, log jam. How you were brought up. You may have been forced as a child to eat vegetables and see it as something undesirable, and you built a perception that plants don't taste good. Another log jam is stress. So much pressure.

We live in a world full of pressure where time matters in all our undertakings, troubled life, and our body pay most of the price.

You have many choices to pick from. If you are a lover of fast food, you need to stop. Fast foods are addictive, and we highly depend on them due to the positive attitude we have towards them. We are obsessed with them such that we cannot live a day without consuming them. When you eat something wrong for you and you say, you don't care. Your thoughts and focus are totally on how delicious and enjoyable it is to be eating the food that you're eating, regardless of how unhealthy it is, and then you have guilt about how those pounds are going on rather than coming off.

Such thoughts occur even when taking tasty food. We may find ourselves eating some food which in reality we know are very dangerous to our health. Chip is a prime example. An individual from a diet class may feel hungry on her way back home and decide to a branch by a fast food joint for some plates of chips. Despite several cautions on the dangers of chips from class lessons, she chooses to eat chips — what a radical idea. Most people have mental disorders making it difficult to stop taking some food even though we understand their repercussions on our bodies, eating chips. An article on this topic claims that most food companies are working hard at night to make fast food more addictive. According to Howard Moskovitz, a consultant in the junk food industry, they put more flavor on junk food to make you come back for more. If the food tastes too good, then we'd have what's called a sensory-specific Satia T then we wouldn't want anymore. So companies have to find just the right balance of flavors. So there's not too much or too little. All they do is to balance the flavors. That balance is called Bliss point.

According to Steven Weatherly, an expert in junk food, Cheetos are the core source of pleasure. They are the specific type of food manufactured by big companies to solely satisfy you and not to add any health benefit to your body. They are designed in such a manner that when you start eating them, it melts on your mouth, making it feels tasty and impressive. They are made to make you go for more. A friend was once a diet, and her boyfriend brought home Cheetos. Yes, she said no. She ended up just having one, and before she knew it, she knew almost the whole thing. Now we understand why the following log in our way is maybe we think we don't like healthy food. Perhaps you don't like healthy food. You want foods that excite your palate to feel alive, be closer to something exciting, but you will not be satisfied.

You'll not reach the maximum point, and perhaps you will not know what to do. Normalizing bad habits make us feel comfortable in our negative thoughts. When you do one negative thing, the effects widely spread. Self-indulgence keeps us wrapped up in this safe place and keeps us inside of ourselves and absorbed by negative thoughts. You know, you do one thing poorly or negatively, it trickles into other areas. It leaves you feeling bad, and you do short to feel better just for the short term, such as impossible diets that you can't keep up with, and then you, you feel worse and worse about yourself and you, you go overboard when you can't keep up. It's a vicious cycle. The primary method of overcoming these key log is to fist, hit the reset button. It might not be easy, strive as much as you can by having an open mind and a positive attitude going forward.

Explore various flavors even if you don't like them. Michael's sister has a negative attitude towards blueberries. She had not consumed any since her childhood and kept telling stories that had no connection to the blueberries' taste. One day Michael made her taste the blueberry, and she loved it. Test your assumptions, test your opinions because you don't know where they came from; such an assumption may be baseless. Despite her premise on blueberries being messy, and she made a try, and she ended up loving it. Open your mind for new ideas. Remember the story of the coy and to keep figuratively throwing yourself in more significant environments, you will stretch out and grow in size. Adopt an attitude of success and stop to fetus thinking and know that your thoughts, perceptions, and behaviors can change. Why not start to look forward to fruit and vegetables, however crazy they sound? You were not born with thoughts you possess today; they are a construct of your mind. They can be challenged.

The following solution calls for changing one's health. Saying a big NO and braking a cycle is all you need — cutting out indulgence. Commit yourself daily, and you'll find it easier to overcome the notion of food industries that want you to be addicted to their food. The third is growth towards what you want and the freedom you desire. This step calls for exceptional consistency. Make your bold step a pattern. This pattern will develop into the desired habit. Unpack your true self through spiritual faith and meditative silence. Strive to become better. Look inside, stop looking for solutions on the outside. Make additional efforts like being more helpful to those that are happy and caring for those that are needy, consistently reach for truth, grace, and peace in your day. Take caution on being a man of the people, and you may be living a fishy life. Finally, systems generate autonomy. We are going to be creating a system together by planning, keeping it simple, embracing balance in your life, and accomplishing these solutions and your goals by following the system to help you prioritize and reinforce consistency in your life.

The best solution to weight loss is a healthy diet and an active body. There could be a reason why doing these two is a problem from your side. The pathway will make the process more holistic and more fun. All may not be your answer, but you must get something from it.

Conclusion

The more that you allow these types of exercises into your life, the more fit and active your mind will be. Having a healthy body is important, but if your mind isn't' healthy first, it will be a much greater struggle.

This process requires willpower, strength, and discipline. Ensure that you are able to incorporate these into your life to see the results you've only been fantasizing about in the past. Pair this with other meditation records as well to get a variety of brain training that will keep you focused on your biggest dreams.

Your attitude can be one of those major things keeping you from reaching your fitness goals. Being on a healthy kick is not necessary for sustainable weight loss.

Losing weight is surely an amazing goal, but it is extremely hard to reach if there is no good motivation to encourage you to keep going.

It absolutely takes some time to reach that ideal weight, both time and effort, and in order to motivate yourself on this journey, the best idea is to embrace positive self-talk.

You need to remind yourself of all of the amazing health benefits of losing weight such as feeling more energized, feeling better about yourself, having better sleep and much more.

In addition to reminding yourself of all of the amazing health benefits of losing weight, another great idea is to keep a success journal where you will write every single step you have taken and succeeded in.

This way you more likely to stay committed to your weight loss journey. In order to boost your commitment, you also need to embrace some positive affirmations and positive self-talk which will keep you going.

Therefore, the succeeding time you look yourself in the mirror, instead of telling yourself I will never be thin and I will just give up, say to yourself this is going to be amazing, losing those five pounds feels great and I will keep going.

Both of these statements are self-talk, but the first one is extremely negative self-talk while the second one is positive self-talk.

These are automatic statements or thoughts to consciously make to yourself. Positive self-talk is an extremely important step as it can influence how you act or how you feel.

Instead of saying to yourself negative statements, embrace positive affirmations that come with some constructive idea.

Once there, your positive self-talk can act as your own personal guardian angel destroying that annoying, destructive devil that has been sitting on your shoulder keeping you from reaching your goals.

If you have battled to stay on the right track in the past, this is mostly due to that annoying negative self-talk which, once there, brings failure, so you are more likely to just give up.

For this reason, say yes to positive self-talk. The most powerful thing about embracing positive self-talk is that those positive affirmations and positive statements you say to yourself tend to stick in your mind, so you are surrounded by positive feelings and thoughts.

In order to start practicing positive self-talk, you need to start listening to what is happening in your mind and recognize your feelings, desires, and fears as these influence your weight loss journey.

The best idea is to keep a weight loss journal where you will write down what you eat that day, how many hours you exercised as well as your feelings and thoughts throughout the day.

If there are some negative statements circling in your head, make sure you write them down. Once you have written them, you need to turn them into affirmations or positive self-talk where instead of I cannot or I will not, you say I can and I will.

As you embrace positive self-talk, you are more likely to stay on the right track. Moreover, as you reshape your negative self-talk into positive self-talk, you also get to change your unique self-definition from a person who cannot achieve something to a person who can achieve anything.

CPSIA information can be obtained
at www.ICGtesting.com
Printed in the USA
BVHW090644270421
605864BV00005B/1101

9 781802 539417